Why Your prenatal Vitamin May Not Be Enough:

The Definitive Guide to Natural Remedies in Pregnancy

By

Tamyra Comeaux

M.D., N.M.D., FACOG

The author, editors, and publisher are not responsible for errors or omissions or for consequences from application of the book, and make no warranty, expressed or implied, in regard to the contents of the book. Any practice described in this book should be applied by the reader in accordance with professional standards of care used in regard to the unique circumstances that may apply in each situation. The reader is advised to always check product information and package inserts for changes and new information regarding dose and contraindications before administering any product.

© 2007 Tamyra Comeaux
All Rights Reserved.

No part of this publication may be reproduced, stored in a retrieval system, or transmitted, in any form or by any means, electronic, mechanical, photocopying, recording, or otherwise, without the written permission of the author.

First published by Dog Ear Publishing
4010 W. 86th Street, Ste H
Indianapolis, IN 46268
www.dogearpublishing.net

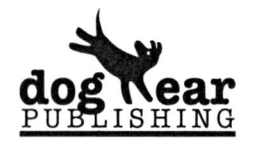

dog ear
PUBLISHING

ISBN: 978-159858-334-2

This book is printed on acid-free paper.

Printed in the United States of America

Table of Contents

Vitamins
- Beta carotene 8
- Biotin 8
- Bromelain 9
- Folic acid 10
- Pantothenic acid 12
- niacin 13
- niacinamide 13
- thiamine 14
- vitamin A 15
- vitamin B-12 16
- vitamin C 17
- vitamin D 19
- vitamin E 20

Minerals
- calcium 21
- chromium 23
- Copper 25
- Iron 25
- magnesium 26
- selenium 30
- zinc 32

Other Nutrients
- Essential fatty acids 33
- flaxseed oil 35
- inositol 35
- lactate 36
- iodine 36
- lactobacillus acidophilus 37
- liver extracts 37
- Sam-E 38

Other botanicals
- bilberry 40
- cranberry 40
- Echinacea 41

elderberry 42
ginger 42
peppermint 43
garlic 44
choline 44

Supplements taken by disease
anxiety 45
anemia 46
allergies 47
asthma 48
carpal tunnel syndrome 49
celiac disease 50
cervical dysplasia 51
common cold 52
constipation 53
depression 55
diabetes 56
eczema 57
fatigue 59
gallstones 60
gastroenteritis 61
headache 61
hemorrhoids 63
herpes 64
homocysteine 66
inflammatory bowel disease .67
insomnia 68
irritable bowel syndrome 69
kidney stones 71
lupus 72
morning sickness 75
obesity 76
preeclampsia 78
premature labor 79
psoriasis 80
rash 81
sciatica 82
smoking dependency 82
Stress 84
stretch marks 85
thyroid disease 86
urinary tract infection 87
recurrent yeast 88

Preface

This book is intended as a reference volume only, not as a medical manual or guide to self-treatment. If you suspect that you have a medical problem, you are urged to seek competent medical help. The information here is intended to help you make informed decisions about the nutritional and herbal supplements you choose, not to substitute for any treatment that may have been prescribed by your physician.

My first advice to an expectant mother is to eat a well-balanced, nutritious diet and be sure to get moderate exercise, fresh air, and plenty of rest. Do not consume junk food, fried food, or too much coffee. Avoid eating rare or undercooked meat, poultry, or fish. Do not eat grilled meats because grilling has been shown to produce carcinogens in meats. Do not smoke, consume alcohol in any form, or use drugs that are not prescribed.

Good nutrition for a female's entire life is the best possible preparation for pregnancy. This is especially true the year or so immediately preceding conception. In a manner of speaking, a baby is nearly one year of age at birth. Many women begin to eat right and take necessary vitamin supplements only after they know they are pregnant. This is weeks or even months too late. The first few weeks of pregnancy are especially crucial to the embryo. Nutrition needs rise during pregnancy, of course. Even the recommended daily allowances are higher. However, many people eat poor diets in general. They then tend to eat more of that same poor diet in an attempt to "eat for two" and get all the nutrition they need from an imbalanced diet. This usually results in weight gain but not necessarily better nutrition for mother and baby. Also, much of the food that we eat may be grown in nutritionally deficient soil. Much of the meat we eat is hormonally and genetically altered. The vegetables can be treated with pesticides or genetically altered. The orthomolecular approach tries to discover such nutrient imbalances and correct them. There is no better time in one's life to start paying attention to one's nutrition than before and during a pregnancy. It was previously thought that one could get all the necessary nutrition from a well-balanced diet. But more and more experts are now encouraging a daily multivitamin, especially during pregnancy. Many people require an intake of certain nutrients far beyond the RDA suggested range, due to their genetic disposition or the environment in which they live.

The reason I am writing this handbook is because I discovered in my private practice in Obstetrics and Gynecology that I cannot write the exact same prenatal vitamin prescription for every single patient. I have discovered that I frequently do have to direct people toward different vitamins, and depending on what a patient tells me, I sometimes have to say, "This vitamin is going to better than that vitamin for you," or "You need to take a different type of supplement in addition." This is because prenatal vitamins, although they are a good start for a pregnancy and a good supplement for a pregnancy, are not sufficient for certain people who have additional stress or medical problems or different things that will be remedied by more or less of a particular nutrient. This handbook is compiled from a number of articles, abstracts, and books about vitamins and supplements. In some cases, the evidence is very good; in other cases, larger numbers of patients are needed to see a clear-cut association. I still recommend the supplement in some cases, because the rationale for studying the supplement in the first place is very good.

Many people are taking over-the-counter remedies or prescription medications before they become pregnant, and then when they become pregnant, they stop taking them or are afraid to take them because they may harm the baby. One must consult with an obstetrician to decide which medicines to continue or discontinue. Sometimes, although I would tell a patient that a particular medicine was reportedly safe to use in pregnancy, the patient would still be reluctant to take it and just suffer through whatever was ailing her. I have often come across articles, or read about studies regarding vitamins treating certain conditions, and have relayed these findings to my patients. I then started to compile fact sheets and made them available for my patients. This book is a result of the fact sheets that have been made available for my patients. As you can imagine, my patients have an impressive collection of vitamins; however, they report that they feel better, are not suffering any medication side effects, and have no guilt feelings regarding "harming" the baby. Vitamins are also an economical way to remedy certain things because almost all of the supplements I recommend can be obtained for less than the cost of an insurance copay.

Patients often ask me what the best prenatal vitamin is. My answer to them is whichever one you like and will take every day. There is a wide range of prenatal vitamins available. The ones over the counter were previously prescription prenatal vitamins and they are all using very similar formulas. There are prescription prenatal vitamins and these formulas are updated on a regular basis. Some of them have more folic acid than the ones over the counter and some of them use a different form of iron that is gentler on the stomach. Some of them have a stool softener included and there are various small differences like that, but in general I encourage patients to find a vitamin they like and can tolerate. If a person takes a vitamin that I think is best but can't keep it down or burps all day or starts having problems with constipation, usually that vitamin gets "forgotten" or is quickly abandoned and that patient ends up taking nothing. I usually give people an assortment of vitamins to try, and some people do very well with all of them and some people like only one particular vitamin. Sometimes different vitamins have a smell that is not agreeable to the patient, and other vitamins have a smell that is very agreeable and makes the vitamin easier to take. I usually encourage people to buy something in a form they will like.

My general philosophy toward any vitamin, whether it's a daily supplement or a prenatal vitamin, is to try to choose one that is dye free and preservative free, just because I don't think prenatal vitamins should include a lot of extra ingredients, things that one is not familiar with.

Try a natural multivitamin, not an artificially colored one. Paint can be nauseating to eat.

Sometimes the directions on the bottle tell you to take supplements with food. Sometimes you might find that the directions say to take the supplements on an empty stomach. Sometimes if people take things on an empty stomach, they get very nauseated or their stomach hurts for a couple of hours. If you find that you have less of a problem when you take it with food or take it before you go to bed, please take your vitamin at these times. Your body knows when it wants to have something. Taking something that is supposed to be good for you and feeling very sick afterward does not help a person maintain the habit of taking that healthy vitamin, so however you can figure out how to get it down and keep it down and not have to think about it five minutes later, that is the way I recommend my patients take their supplements. Also, I encourage a lot of my patients to take iron, but I find that if they go to the store and buy the least expensive form of iron, which is usually ferrous sulfate iron, these are the people who come back with the most complaints, and usually by the time I see them again they tell me they abandoned those supplements within a week of beginning to take them. Iron is better taken with vitamin C. There are some formulations, by prescription, where they can be taken with vitamin C. Feosol, which is available over the counter, is an easier-to-absorb form of iron; or one can use carbonyl iron, which is in many prescription prenatal vitamins. Ferrous fumarate and ferrous gluconate are also available over the counter.

Some people have religious restrictions on what they can eat and need a kosher vitamin or a vitamin without gelatin, and I direct the patient toward these types of vitamins also or I can make recommendations when requested.

Pregnancy is a time when nutrition is doubly important, and I think of a prenatal vitamin as extra insurance. The baby gets everything it needs and the mother retains everything she needs, if the baby does end up depleting her stores of particular vitamins. Also during pregnancy, people like to avoid taking multiple over-the-counter and prescription medications. People frequently stop taking medications they were previously taking, but they still have problems like headaches, depression and stress, and frequent colds. There are additional vitamin supplements that can help make these other medications less crucial.

This book is organized as follows:

1. A description of different types of vitamins and their uses.
2. A section for each particular disease or pregnancy state in which additional supplements are recommended.
3. Parameters listed for the maximum amount of each particular vitamin that can be taken. Sometimes people might have three different problems and want to take vitamins from three different sections, but people must be careful to ensure they are not taking over the limit of each type of supplement. In general, it would be difficult to cause a problem taking vitamins and minerals, but still people can have uncomfortable side effects such as diarrhea, constipation, headaches, and other, more serious complications by taking too many vitamins. Therefore, people should be careful to add up the amount of certain supplements and make sure they are not taking too much.

Vitamins in Prenatal Vitamins

Beta-carotene

Beta-carotene is found in many prenatal vitamins. Beta carotene is converted into vitamin A. The conversion of beta-carotene to vitamin A is dependent on several factors including protein status, thyroid hormones, zinc, and vitamin C. Beta-carotene, in general, does not lead to vitamin A toxicity. It is naturally found in fruits and vegetables, especially green vegetables, carrots, apricots, mangos, yams, squash, tomatoes, and plums. Beta-carotene is safe during pregnancy and lactation and has no known overdosage risks.

Biotin

Biotin is another vitamin found in prenatal vitamins. It is more frequently found in prenatal vitamins obtained from health food stores. It is occasionally in prescription prenatal vitamins. It is good for building strong nails and healthy hair. It is a member of the B vitamin family. People with a biotin deficiency may exhibit dry, scaly skin, nausea, and loss of appetite. Biotin supplementation has been shown to enhance insulin activity and improve the utilization of blood sugar. If you've had problems with your sugar in the past or have been a gestational diabetic in the past, make sure you have a vitamin that does have biotin in it. If you have brittle nails, make sure your prenatal vitamin has biotin in it. Human studies have shown that biotin supplementation, up to 2.5 mg/day, can produce a 25% increase in the thickness of the nail plate in patients diagnosed with brittle nails of unknown cause, and up to 91% of patients taking this dosage experienced definite improvement.

Individuals with diabetes should use caution when using high dosages of biotin that is greater than 4 milligrams, because it may produce reductions of blood sugars that require changes in the dosages of insulin or other medications. Biotin is extremely safe and no side effects have been reported. Eight hundred micrograms of Biotin in a prenatal vitamin would be a good amount to expect. This is more than twice the recommended daily value, and it is safe during pregnancy and lactation.

Bromelain

For a pregnant woman, it is most useful as a digestive aid and for respiratory tract infections. Bromelain refers to a group of sulphur-containing proteolytic enzymes or proteases, which are enzymes that digest protein obtained from the pineapple plant. One could eat pineapple to obtain this particular enzyme. Commercial bromelain is usually derived from the stem, which differs from the bromelain derived from eating the fruit. Bromelain was introduced as a therapeutic agent in 1957, and since that time more than 200 scientific papers on its therapeutic applications have appeared in the medical literature. Bromelain is one of the most popular natural agents in use because of its ability to impact many aspects of inflammation. It is used predominantly in cases of injuries, brain strain, arthritis, recovery from surgery, and other inflammatory conditions. However, it is also used as a digestive aid and in infections, particularly respiratory tract infections.

Bromelain exerts several beneficial effects in respiratory tract infections such as sinusitis, bronchitis, and even pneumonia. For example, in addition to its antibiotic activity, bromelain suppresses cough and reduces the viscosity of sputum. Bromelain is also helpful in acute sinusitis. Bromelain is available primarily in tablets and capsules. If you are allergic to pineapple, do not use bromelain. Copper and iron deactivate bromelain, so it should be taken at a separate time as nutrient supplements containing these two, and magnesium activates it, so it can be taken at the same time as the magnesium supplement.

If you are using bromelain as a digestive agent, it can be taken with food, but if you are using it for another purpose, such as for an upper respiratory infection, it is recommended that it be taken at a different time than food. The typical dosage of bromelain is 250–750 mg three times a day, between meals. Overdosage is virtually non-toxic. Dosages up to 10 grams/kilogram of body weight were not associated with any deaths. Possible side effects at high doses (greater than 2 grams would be a high dose) include symptoms such as nausea, vomiting, or diarrhea. Bromelain is considered safe during pregnancy and lactation.

Folic Acid

An important message from the March of Dimes:

"Folic acid is needed for cell growth. It is particularly critical during the earliest weeks, when a baby's organs are forming. Adequate intake of the folic acid before and in early pregnancy may reduce the risk of birth defects in the brain and spinal cord. The average American gets only 285 mcg of folic acid a day—far short of the 400 mcg minimum that is recommended. Over 50% of all neural tube defects may be prevented if all women of childbearing age would consume 400 mcg of folic acid daily beginning one month before conception and 800 mcg throughout pregnancy." For more information about having a healthy baby, call the March of Dimes at 1-888-modimes or go to www.marchofdimes.com.

Folic acid is a very important vitamin and a prenatal vitamin. Over-the-counter prenatal vitamins will usually have about 800 micrograms of this supplement. Prescription prenatal vitamins will have 1 milligram. This is a very small difference, and 800 micrograms is sufficient for most people. However, anyone who has had a child with a neural tube defect in the past, or anyone who has a history of seizure disorder or is on seizure medication, should get a prescription from her physician and would usually be taking up to 4 mg per day of this vitamin. Without folic acid, cells do not divide properly. Folic acid usually functions together with Vitamin B-12 in many body processes. Deficiency of folic acid during pregnancy has been linked to several birth defects and is also being linked to depression, atherosclerosis, and osteoporosis. Folic acid reduces body concentrations of homocysteine, which has been implicated in a variety of conditions including atherosclerosis and osteoporosis. Homocysteine is thought to promote atherosclerosis by directly damaging the artery as well as reducing the integrity of the vessel wall. In osteoporosis, elevated homocysteine levels lead to a defective bone matrix by interfering with the proper formation of collagen. In pregnant women who have had miscarriages in the past, I frequently measure a hormone called methyltetrahydrofolate reductase. People who have a problem with this gene do not metabolize folic acid properly, and this leads to a high incidence of homocysteine in their bloodstream, which leads to the problems I've just mentioned. In people who do have a deficiency of this gene, I do prescribe extra folic acid.

Cervical dysplasia is an abnormal condition of the cells of the cervix. It is generally regarded as a precancerous lesion and has risk factors similar to those of cervical cancer. It is quite probable that many abnormal pap smears reflect folate deficiency rather than true dysplasia, especially in women who are pregnant or are taking oral contraceptives, because estrogens antagonize folic acid. Folic acid supplementation, up to 10 mg/day, has resulted in improvement or normalization of pap smears in patients with cervical dysplasia in clinical studies. At this time, the upper limit of folic acid in pregnancy is 1 milligram. I do not recommend that a patient who is pregnant take that particular amount of folic acid that is 10 times the amount in a prescription vitamin; however, I would have that patient ensure that she is taking the maximum amount possible.

Folic acid exerts a mild antidepressant affect, presumably via its function as a methyl donor, which helps increase serotonin levels in the brain. Folic acid supplementation in depressed patients taking antidepressants drugs such as Prozac (fluoxetine is the generic name), was found to enhance the antidepressant actions of these drugs, and numerous studies have demonstrated the benefit of folic acid supplementation in pregnancy beginning either before conception or very early in the pregnancy and continuing throughout in preventing a type of birth defect known as neural tube defect, otherwise known as spina bifida.

Folic acid is available as folate and as folinic acid. In order to use folic acid, the body must convert it to folinic acid. Therefore, supplying the body with folinic acid allows it to bypass this process. Some prenatal vitamins have metafolin in order to make the folate in the prenatal vitamin more bioavailable. Folic acid supplementation should always include vitamin B-12 supplementation because folic acid can mask an underlying vitamin B-12 deficiency. This is why the FDA restricts the amount of folic acid available in dietary supplements to 800 micrograms. The danger is that while the folic acid will reverse the pernicious anemia caused by the B-12 deficiency, it will not prevent or reverse the related neurological symptoms. High doses of folic acid may cause increased flatulence, nausea, and loss of appetite, but the level of folic acid that causes this is 5000–10000 micrograms daily, whereas most prenatal vitamins contain one-tenth this amount. No side effects have been reported at lower dosages. Even people on prophylaxis for spina bifida at the 4000-microgram dose should not have these side effects. Folic acid supplements are generally better absorbed than the folic acid naturally present in foods. There are no known overdosage effects for folic acid, and it is safe for pregnant and breastfeeding women.

Pantothenic Acid

Pantothenic acid, or vitamin B-5, is available most often in capsules and tablets as calcium pantothenate. High dosages of pantothenic acid may inhibit the absorption of biotin. Pantothenic acid is generally regarded as safe during pregnancy and lactation; however, because its effects during these times have not been sufficiently evaluated, it should not be used by pregnant or lactating women at dosages greater than 100 milligrams unless specifically directed to do so by a physician. Pantothenic acid is not available in some prenatal vitamins. When present in prescription prenatal vitamins it is usually between 6 and 10 milligrams. Prenatal vitamins in the health food store may have up to 25 milligrams.

Pantothenic vitamin is known as the anti-stress vitamin. It plays a role in the production of adrenal hormones and the formation of antibodies, aids in vitamin utilization and helps to convert fats, carbohydrates, and proteins into energy. It is required by all cells in the body and is concentrated in the organs. It is also involved in the production of neurotransmitters. This vitamin is an essential element of coenzyme A, a vital body chemical involved in many necessary metabolic functions. Pantothenic acid is also a stamina enhancer and prevents certain forms of anemia. It is needed for normal functioning of the gastrointestinal tract and may be helpful in treating depression and anxiety. A deficiency of pantothenic acid may cause fatigue, headache, nausea, and tingling in the hands. Pantothenic acid is also needed for proper functioning of the adrenal glands.

Sources. The following foods contain pantothenic acid: beef, brewer's yeast, eggs, fresh vegetables, kidney, legumes, liver, mushrooms, nuts, pork, jelly, saltwater fish, and whole wheat.

Niacin

Niacin, or vitamin B3, is found in some prenatal vitamins. The amount of niacin in a prenatal vitamin is generally adequate when present, and I do not advise people to buy additional supplement of this during pregnancy. It is usually found in the form of niacin amide. Niacin can be used to lower cholesterol; however, I do not recommend that pregnant women take the dosages required for this effect during pregnancy. In doses greater than 50 mg, niacin can cause flushing of the skin. Niacin is safe during pregnancy and lactation at dosages below 35 milligrams. According to the National Academy of Sciences, Dietary Reference Intakes: A Risk Assessment Model for Establishing Upper Intake Levels for Nutrients. "Niacin is safe up to the dose 100 mg," according to Michael Murray, N.D., in *The pill book Guide to Natural Medicines*.

Niacinamide

Niacinamide is also known as nicotinamide. It is a form of vitamin B3 that has different effects than niacin. The amount of niacinamide in a prenatal vitamin is generally adequate when present and I do not advise people to buy additional supplements of this during pregnancy because this is the form usually found in prenatal vitamins in the amount of 20 mg. The maximum recommended amount in pregnancy is 30 mg. This can be used to treat osteoarthritis, rheumatoid arthritis, and diabetes, but in much higher doses than those allowed in pregnancy.

Riboflavin

Riboflavin is also known as vitamin B-2. Riboflavin deficiency is characterized by cracking of the lips and corners of the mouth, inflamed tongue, visual disturbances such as sensitivity to light and loss of visual acuity, cataract formation, burning and itching of the eyes, mouth, lips, and tongue and other signs of disorders of the mucus membranes. Riboflavin supplementation is used specifically in cataracts, prevention of migraine headaches, and sickle cell anemia. I do recommend that my patients with migraine headaches take riboflavin but in the form of a B-complex vitamin, and people with sickle cell trait also benefit from B-complex vitamin supplementation. No side effects of riboflavin are known, even at higher dosages, but when people with migraines were studied, high doses, over 400 milligrams per day, produced diarrhea and increased urinary frequency in two patients. Taking riboflavin with food increases its absorption, and riboflavin is necessary to convert vitamin B-6 to its active form; for this reason, when I want a patient to take a particular B vitamin, I recommend taking a B-complex vitamin. Most of the B vitamins are found together in foods and work very well together. The dosage of riboflavin in a prenatal vitamin is generally about 10 milligrams or less. The capacity of the human gastrointestinal tract to absorb riboflavin might be less than 20 milligrams in single oral dose. No overdose of riboflavin has been recorded. Riboflavin is considered safe during pregnancy and lactation.

Thiamin

Thiamin is vitamin B-1 and was the first B vitamin discovered, hence its designation is Vitamin B-1. Thiamin is essential for proper energy production in every cell of the body but especially in the heart and brain. Severe Thiamin deficiency was discovered as the cause of a syndrome known as beri beri. Symptoms include mental confusion, muscle wasting, fluid retention, high blood pressure, difficulty walking, and heart disturbances. Pregnant women frequently report that they can't retain information as well or think as well, especially as the pregnancy progresses I encourage a B-complex supplement in this case. Also people who are complaining of fluid retention could benefit from an additional B-complex. Thiamin appears to be safe during pregnancy and lactation at dosage levels less than 100 mg daily. Thiamin is not associated with any toxicity. The usual amount of thiamin in a prenatal vitamin is 3 milligrams. The dose of riboflavin in a prenatal vitamin is usually 3.4 milligrams. The formulations in health food stores can contain up to 10 milligrams. The recommended daily allowance for thiamin is 1.5 milligrams and 1.6 milligrams in lactating women. For riboflavin it is 1.4 milligrams in pregnant women and 1.6 milligrams in lactating women.

Vitamin A

Vitamin A was the first fat-soluble vitamin to be discovered. Vitamin A is necessary for proper visual function, immune system activity, growth and development, and reproduction and integrity of the skin and mucous membranes. Vitamin A is necessary to mount an effective immune system response. Individuals deficient in vitamin A are more susceptible to infectious diseases in general but especially viral infections. Do not supplement with more than 5000 international units of vitamin A per day if you are pregnant or at risk of becoming pregnant. Do not supplement with vitamin A without consulting a physician if you suffer from cirrhosis of the liver, hepatitis, or any other serious liver disorder. At recommended levels in people with normal liver function, vitamin A is not associated with any side effects. Because high doses of vitamin A during pregnancy can cause birth defects, women of childbearing age should not supplement with more than 5000 international units of vitamin A per day. Beta carotene is a suitable, nontoxic alternative. The same warning applies during lactation. Most prenatal vitamin supplements include their vitamin A in the form of beta carotene, which can be supplemented above 5000 international units without consequence. Almost all prenatal vitamins use beta carotene exclusively as their source of vitamin A. There are also a couple of prenatal vitamins that do not contain vitamin A at all. Because it is a fat-soluble vitamin that is stored in the body, it is not common in this country for a person to have a deficiency of vitamin A. I rarely recommend vitamin A supplements above what is in a prenatal vitamin or in the diet for pregnant women for any condition.

Vitamin B-6

Vitamin B-6, pyridoxine, is an extremely important B vitamin for which a deficiency is characterized by depression and/or anemia. In patients with depression and eczema, I do recommend extra supplements of this vitamin. It is also very important in pregnant women who are nauseated. B-6 supplementation is also helpful in cases of carpal tunnel syndrome but may take as long as three months to produce a benefit. Unfortunately, many pregnant women get this at the end of their pregnancy. Excessive dosages of vitamin B-6 can lead to significant toxicity, noted as tingling sensations in the feet, loss of muscle coordination, and degeneration of nerve tissue. Usually these symptoms are seen at a dosage of 500 milligrams per day but can be seen at dosages as low as 150 milligrams per day. Dosages should be limited to about 50 milligrams per day. If a person takes more than 50 milligrams per day, the dosages should be spread out through the day. During the first trimester, actually 25 milligrams three times per day would be a dose at which one could expect some improvement, and this dosage is safe. The upper limit of vitamin B-6 for a pregnant woman daily is 100 milligrams.

B-6 is of special concern for both pregnant and lactating women because studies have shown that the requirement for this nutrient increases at these times. Moreover, studies have found that pregnant women consume only 50% of the recommended daily allowance during the last month of pregnancy and that breastfeeding women consume only 60% of the recommended daily allowance after delivery. B-6 supplementation has been found to reduce the nausea and vomiting during pregnancy. Another study found that Apgar scores (which are a measure of a newborn's health) were significantly better for infants of mothers who took an amount several times the recommended daily allowance of B-6 than for those who took an amount close the recommended daily allowance. Adequate levels of B-6 are also vital in lactating women because of the previously mentioned association of B-6 deficiency with convulsions and irritability in some infants.

The bioavailability of B6 from food sources is limited. "The amount of B6 found in foods does not necessarily represent the amount of the vitamin available to humans" as reported in the *Journal of Nutrition* in 1983.

Vitamin B-12

Vitamin B-12 is found in significant quantities in animal foods. The richest sources are liver and kidney followed by eggs, fish, cheese, and meat. Therefore it is very important that vegetarians supplement their diets with vitamin B-12. Unlike other water-soluble nutrients, vitamin B-12 is stored in the liver, kidney, and other body tissues. As a result, signs and symptoms of vitamin B-12 deficiency may not show themselves until after five to six years of poor dietary intake. Vitamin B-12 deficiency can produce symptoms such as numbness, a pins-and-needles sensation, or a burning feeling in the feet as well as impaired mental function. In the elderly, a deficiency can mimic Alzheimer's disease. A vitamin B-12 deficiency can also result in a smooth, beefy-looking red tongue. Diarrhea is another symptom.

It is possible to inject vitamin B-12 for the treatment of anemia and B-12 deficiency, in most healthy pregnant women injection is not required because the oral administration of an appropriate dosage has been shown to produce results as good as those of injectable preparations. Vitamin B-12 deficiency can cause depression, and correcting such a deficiency usually results in a dramatic improvement in mood. Certain drugs can interfere with the absorption or utilization of vitamin B-12, such as some antibiotics, Aldomet, Tagamet, glucophage, Pepcid, Prevacid, Prilosec, and Zantac. So for anyone experiencing heartburn and taking over-the-counter antacids, usually the amount of B-12 in the prenatal vitamin is adequate, but I recommend taking these medications at least two hours apart; however, if the person is having any other problems, such as with anemia or depression, I recommend an additional B-Complex supplement. Vitamin B-12 supplementation is generally regarded as safe during pregnancy and lactation and there are no known side effects with an overdose of vitamin B-12.

Vitamin C

The primary function of vitamin C is the manufacture of collagen. It is also critical to immune function and in the absorption and utilization of other nutritional factors. Since 1973 there have been 11 clinical studies of vitamin C supplementation for asthma. Seven of these studies showed significant improvements in respiratory measures and asthma symptoms as a result of supplementing the diet with 1–2 grams of vitamin C daily. The upper limit that is recommended in pregnant women is 2 grams. Claims have been made about the role of vitamin C in the prevention and treatment of the common cold. Since 1970 there have been 20 double-blind studies designed to assess what role vitamin C can play in the common cold. In the majority of the studies vitamin C supplementation produced a decrease in either duration or symptom severity. Analysis of all studies indicates that vitamin C at a dosage of 1–6 grams daily decreased the duration of the cold episodes by 21%. This could also be why it helps asthmatics; this is my personal thought. Frequently people who get flu or colds or some sort of virus have their asthma exacerbated. So if people are supplementing to make sure that they don't catch a cold, then their asthma will not deteriorate.

Vitamin C supplementation also appears to be indicated in preventing at least two complications of pregnancy: preeclampsia and premature rupture of the fetal membranes. Preeclampsia is a serious condition of pregnancy associated with elevations in blood pressure, fluid retention, and loss of protein in the urine. Free radical damage to the lining of blood vessels is known to play a key role in the development of preeclampsia. Antioxidants are critically involved in the protection of the vascular endothelium. Low antioxidant levels including vitamin C have been shown to be a predisposing factor in preeclampsia. Premature rupture of the fetal membranes is one of the major contributors of infant morbidity and mortality. The cause of premature rupture of membranes is unclear but may in some cases be due to low levels of vitamin C. In one study, these subjects have significantly lower levels of vitamin C in the amniotic fluid. Vitamin C supplementation at daily doses greater than 500 milligrams is not advised for people on hemodialysis, which is rare in pregnant women; or for those who suffer from recurrent kidney stones, which is not rare in pregnant women; or for severe kidney disease or gout, because higher dosages may possibly increase kidney stone formation in these patients.

Vitamin C is extremely safe in most people, but diarrhea and intestinal distension, or gas, are the most common complaints at higher dosage levels. People who do experience these symptoms while supplementing with vitamin C in pregnancy should decrease their dosage to approximately half and remain at this dosage if it is tolerated.

There are possible drug interactions between certain medications and vitamin C. Vitamin C may increase the absorption of aluminum from aluminum-containing antacids such as Maalox and Mylanta; therefore, a person should take vitamin C at least two hours after taking one of these products. Vitamin C also increases the absorption of iron and copper. It may also interfere with the blood test for vitamin B-12. If a person is on iron supplementation for any reason, I advise her to take vitamin C with it. Most of the prescription iron today is formulated to come with vitamin C, folic acid, and B-12. Anyone taking over-the-counter iron should take vitamin C at the same time or at least drink orange juice to enhance the absorption of iron. In healthy individuals a daily dosage of 100–500 milligrams is believed to be sufficient; however, higher dosages may be necessary in certain health conditions such as asthma, diabetes, cataracts, and the common cold. In these health conditions the dosage ranges from 500–2000 milligrams per day.

Vitamin D

It is well known that vitamin D stimulates the absorption of calcium. Because vitamin D can be produced in our body by the action of sunlight on the skin, many experts consider it more of a hormone than a vitamin. Vitamin D deficiency results in rickets in children and osteomalacia in adults. Rickets is characterized by an inability to calcify the bone matrix. This results in softening of the skull bones, bowing of the legs, spinal curvature, and increased joint size. This disease is extremely rare. Vitamin D deficiency is now most often seen in elderly people who do not get any sunlight, particularly those in nursing homes. The consequences are joint pain and lack of bone strength and density.

Vitamin D supplementation alone and in combination with calcium has been shown to reduce osteoporosis and hip fractures. In one study using vitamin D-3 alone, it was shown that supplementation with vitamin D reduced the annual rate of hip fractures by nearly 60 percent. Vitamin D is generally well tolerated with no side effects at the recommended dosages. Phenobarbital and mineral oil both interfere with the absorption and/or metabolism of vitamin D. Corticosteroids, such as prednisone, increase the need for vitamin D. Olestra, which is a fat substitute, as well as sources of dietary fiber and Pectin may decrease the absorption of vitamin D. The recommended daily allowance of vitamin D is 200–400 international units daily. There has not been a role found for supplementation greater than 400 international units in most adults and young children. Vitamin D has the potential to cause toxicity. Dosages greater than 1000 international units per day are usually not recommended. Toxicity is characterized by increased blood concentration of calcium, deposition of calcium into internal organs, and kidney stones. Because vitamin D is a fat-soluble vitamin and can be stored in the body, it should not be taken during pregnancy and lactation at greater than recommended levels. In prenatal vitamins the dose of vitamin D is 400 international units.

Vitamin E

Vitamin E functions primarily as an antioxidant, protecting against damage to the cell membranes. Without vitamin E, the cells of the body would be quite susceptible to damage. Severe vitamin E deficiency is quite rare but there are four major groups among whom low levels of vitamin E are common: (1) people with a fat malabsorption syndrome such as celiac disease, cystic fibrosis, and post-gastrectomy syndrome; (2) premature infants; (3) people with hereditary disorders of blood cells, such as sickle cell disease and thalassemia; and (4) hemodialysis patients. Symptoms of vitamin E deficiency in adults include nerve damage, muscle weakness, poor coordination, involuntary movement of the eyes, and breaking of red blood cells leading to anemia. Vitamin E may increase bleeding tendency and should not be used for at least one week prior to any elective surgery. The amount of vitamin E found in a prenatal vitamin is generally 30 international units, which is well below the level at which a person would bleed. The range found in prenatal vitamins is between 30 and 100 international units. The upper limit in pregnancy is 1000 international units. Vitamin E supplementation is generally regarded as safe during pregnancy and lactation. Although vitamin E is a fat-soluble vitamin, it has an excellent safety record. Dosages high as 3,200 international units daily for periods up to two years have not shown any unfavorable side effects. Detailed safety assessments have also shown that vitamin E supplementation is extremely safe.

Minerals Commonly Used in Pregnancy and Lactation

Calcium

Calcium is the most abundant mineral in the body. It constitutes 1.5–2% of the total body weight, with more than 99% of the calcium being present in bones. In addition to its major function in building and maintaining bones and teeth, calcium is also important in the activities of many enzymes in the body. The contraction of muscles, release of neurotransmitters, regulation of heartbeat, and clotting of blood are all dependent on calcium. Population studies have suggested a link between high blood pressure and a low dietary intake of calcium. It appears that calcium supplementation, 1–1.5 grams per day, is most likely to produce effective reductions in blood pressure in Afro-Americans, people who are salt-sensitive, and elderly patients.

Another condition associated with high blood pressure that may respond to or be prevented by calcium supplementation is preeclampsia, which is a serious condition of pregnancy associated with elevations in blood pressure, fluid retention, and loss of protein in the urine. Early studies in pregnancy women suggested that a low calcium intake was a major risk factor for hypertension and preeclampsia during pregnancy. The results from clinical studies have now demonstrated that pregnant women who receive calcium supplementation during pregnancy have a reduced risk of hypertension and preelcampsia. I highly recommend that all of my patients with chronic hypertension and who have had a history of preeclampsia in a previous pregnancy or those at risk of preecampsia in a current pregnancy, such as teenagers, diabetics, and people who are of advanced maternal age, supplement with 1000–1500 milligrams of calcium daily. Most prenatal vitamins have approximately 150 milligrams of calcium, and I recommend that people take an additional supplement. Usually, over-the-counter calcium supplements come in either 500 or 600 milligrams, and I recommend that people take two of these daily so that they will be getting between 1000 and 1200 milligrams of calcium. Usually this calcium also comes with vitamin D. Sometimes the calcium can also come with magnesium. There are already 400 international units of vitamin D in a prenatal vitamin. People taking an additional over-the-counter calcium supplement are usually getting additional vitamin D. As previously mentioned, up to 1000 international units of vitamin D is okay. It is important to make sure that a dosage of 1000 international units of vitamin D is not exceeded.

I also recommend calcium for people who are suffering from leg cramps. For people who are already taking a prenatal vitamin with vitamin D included, I recommend a calcium supplement that does not have vitamin D. Many patients who have heartburn are already on Tums; if you are taking Tums for heartburn, you should be careful to total your calcium intake to not exceed 1500 milligrams of calcium. Calcium supplements are available in capsules, tablets, chewable wafers, liquids, and powders. The most widely used form is calcium carbonate. Oyster shell calcium, dolomite, and bone meal are forms of calcium but at one a time they reportedly contained high levels of lead and other impurities, and I do not prefer these forms during pregnancy. Calcium supplements are generally well-tolerated at dosages lower than 2000 milligrams. Higher dosages may increase the risk for kidney stones and soft tissue calcification; however, neither of these two conditions has been conclusively linked to calcium supplementation. Aluminum-containing antacids are known to ultimately lead to an increase in bone breakdown and calcium excretion. Anti-ulcer drugs, such as Tagamet, Zantac, Pepcid, and Prilosec, which are all over-the-counter, can decrease calcium absorption because they block the output of hydrochloric acid. Thyroid hormones such as Levoxyl and Synthroid should not be taken within two hours of calcium supplements because the calcium may decrease their absorption and effectiveness. Calcium supplementation may also decrease the effectiveness of Dilantin. If you are taking one of these drugs, please consult your physician before taking a calcium supplement. Absorption of calcium carbonate is enhanced when taken with food. Calcium supplementation is safe and actually recommended in pregnancy and breastfeeding. It is especially important that pregnant and lactating women receive enough calcium. Overdosage of calcium is rare. Early signs of an overdose are severe constipation, dryness of the mouth, headache, increased thirst, irritability, loss of appetite, mental depression, and unusual tiredness or weakness.

Chromium

Chromium functions in the body as a key constituent of the glucose tolerance factor. Chromium works closely with insulin in facilitating the uptake of glucose into the cells. Without chromium, insulin's action is blocked and blood sugar levels are elevated. Chromium's key beneficial effect is to help insulin work properly. Nearly twenty controlled studies have a demonstrated positive effect for chromium in the treatment of diabetes. In clinical studies, in non-insulin dependent diabetic patients, supplementing the diet with chromium has been shown to decrease fasting glucose levels, improve glucose tolerance, lower insulin levels, and decrease total cholesterol and triglyceride levels while increasing HDL cholesterol levels. The typical dosage recommendation for chromium is 200–600 micrograms per day. Chromium is considered safe in pregnant and lactating women. Individuals with diabetes need to be aware that chromium supplementation may alter insulin or drug requirements. Please consult your physician to discuss proper monitoring of blood sugar levels before taking chromium. Chromium is not available in all prenatal vitamins, and the patients to whom I recommend an additional chromium supplement are those who have excessive weight gain, gestational diabetes, history of hypoglycemia, and are diabetics. I usually recommend about 200 micrograms per day in these instances.

Chromium is necessary for regulating your body's blood sugar levels and stimulates the synthesis of protein in the fetus' developing tissues. Everyone needs at least 50 micrograms daily, which is a fairly easy amount to get through your diet. If you eat a slice of whole wheat bread, one apple and three ounces of chicken, you'd be just over the recommended daily allowance. The best food sources are whole grain breads and cereals, wheat germ, asparagus, and brewers yeast. Others include: one slice of American cheese, which has 48 micrograms; one tablespoon of peanut butter, which has 41 micrograms; one cup of boiled spinach, which has 36 micrograms; 3 ounces of broiled, skinless chicken, which has 22 micrograms; 1 cup of button mushrooms, which has 20 micrograms; one slice of whole grain bread, which has 16 micrograms; and one medium apple, which has 15 micrograms.

Many prescription prenatal vitamins do not contain any chromium. The daily allowance for pregnant women is 30 micrograms, but some evidence suggests that chromium deficiency might be relatively common; however, this has not been proven, and the matter is greatly complicated by the fact that we lack a good test to identify chromium deficiency. Severe chromium deficiency has been seen only in hospitalized individuals receiving nutrition intravenously. Symptoms include problems with blood sugar control that cannot be corrected by insulin alone. The most concentrated sources of chromium are brewer's yeast and calf liver. Two ounces of brewer's yeast or four ounces of calf liver provide between 50 and 60 micrograms of chromium. Calcium carbonate interferes with the absorption of chromium. The dosage of chromium used in studies ranges from 200–1000 micrograms daily; however, there may be risks in the higher dosages of chromium.

Moderately strong evidence supports the use of chromium for diabetes. In a recent double-blind, placebo-controlled study, 180 people with type-2 diabetes were given placebo 200 micrograms of chromium picolinate daily or a higher dosage of chromium picolinate 1000 micrograms daily. Individuals taking 1000 micrograms showed marked improvements in blood sugar levels. Lesser but still significant benefits were also seen in the 200 microgram group but not in the placebo group. One placebo-controlled study of 30 women with pregnancy-related diabetes found that supplementation with chromium at a dosage of 4 or 8 micrograms of chromium picolinate for each kilogram of body weight significantly improved blood sugar control. Chromium might also be helpful for treating diabetes caused by corticosteroid treatment. Another small, double-blind trial found that chromium improved the body's response to insulin among overweight people at risk of developing diabetes. The evidence is mixed on whether chromium is an effective aid in weight loss. This is not a use I would find for chromium during pregnancy anyway. Although the precise upper limit of safe chromium intake is not known, it is believed that chromium is safe when taken at a dosage of 50–200 micrograms daily. Side effects appear to be rare. However, chromium is a heavy metal and might conceivably build up and cause problems if taken to excess. There was one report of kidney and liver damage in a person who took 1200–2400 micrograms of chromium for several months. In another report, as low as 600 micrograms for six weeks was enough to cause damage. Such problems appear to be quite rare, and it is possible that these individuals already had health problems that predisposed them to such a reaction. The risk of chromium toxicity is believed to be higher in individuals who already have liver or kidney disease. A pregnant woman should consult with her physician before she decides to supplement with chromium, and I recommend that until further studies are performed, supplementation with 200 micrograms or less should be the limit.

Copper

Copper is the third most abundant essential trace element in the human body after iron and zinc. The highest concentration of copper is found in the brain and liver. Copper is required for proper iron absorption and utilization. Therefore, copper deficiency can result in iron deficiency anemia. Copper deficiency manifests itself in rupture of blood vessels, osteoporosis and bone and joint abnormalities. Many prenatal vitamins do contain the RDA of copper, and I rarely advise people to buy an additional copper supplement to take. There are usually about 2 milligrams of copper in a prenatal vitamin when present at all. This amount of copper is considered safe during pregnancy and lactation. The upper-limit safe level is 10 milligrams.

Iron

Iron is critical to human life. It plays the central role in the hemoglobin molecule of red blood cells, functioning to transport oxygen from the lungs to the body's tissues and transport carbon dioxide from the tissues to the lungs. Iron also functions in several key enzymes involved in energy production and metabolism, including DNA synthesis. Iron deficiency is the most common nutrient deficiency in the United States. Groups at very high risk for iron deficiency are teenage girls and pregnant women. Studies have found evidence of iron deficiency in as many as 30–50% of individuals in these groups. Almost all prenatal vitamins have iron in them. Some people do not tolerate iron very well and get very constipated and have diarrhea and gas. There is a prenatal vitamin at GNC that is formulated without iron for people who are otherwise unable to tolerate a prenatal vitamin with iron. Most people are on a prenatal vitamin with iron, and for patients who are anemic I do frequently prescribe an additional iron supplement, usually one that contains vitamin C. Iron deficiency may be due to an increased iron requirement, decreased dietary intake, diminished iron absorption or utilization, blood loss, or a combination of factors. Increased requirements for iron occur during the growth spurts of infancy and adolescence and during pregnancy and lactation. Currently the vast majority of pregnant women are routinely given iron supplements during pregnancy because the dramatically increased need for iron cannot usually be met through diet alone. The most common side effects of iron are mild gastrointestinal irritation, constipation or diarrhea, and nausea. Antacids such as Tagamet, Zantac, Pepcid, and Prilosec can decrease iron absorption.

Thyroid hormones such as Levoxyl and Synthroid should not be taken within two hours of iron supplements because the iron may decrease their absorption and effectiveness. Calcium, magnesium, and zinc can also interfere with iron absorption. Vitamin C enhances iron absorption. For people with iron deficiency, the usual recommendation is 37 milligrams of elemental iron twice daily between meals. Most prenatal vitamins contain between 27 and 40 milligrams of iron. It may come in the form of ferrous fumarate or carbonyl iron.

Magnesium

Magnesium is second only to potassium in terms of concentration within the individual cells of the body. The functions of magnesium primarily revolve around its ability to activate many enzymes.

Magnesium deficiency is extremely common in Americans, particularly in the geriatric population and in women during the premenstrual period. Deficiency is often secondary to factors that reduce absorption or increase secretions of magnesium such as high calcium intake, alcoholism, surgery, diuretics, liver disease, kidney disease, and oral contraceptive use. The signs and symptoms of magnesium deficiency include fatigue, mental confusion, irritability, weakness, heart disturbances, problems in nerve conduction and muscle contraction, muscle cramps, loss of appetite, insomnia, and a predisposition to stress.

There is considerable evidence from population studies that a high intake of magnesium is associated with lower blood pressure. Because of this evidence, researchers began investigating the effect of magnesium supplementation in the treatment of high blood pressure. The results from double-blind studies have been mixed. Some of the studies have shown a very good blood pressure lowering effect, whereas others have not. The degree of blood pressure reduction with magnesium is generally modest, that is, less than 10 millimeters of mercury for both systolic and diastolic measures.

For diabetes, magnesium is known to play a central role in the secretion and action of insulin. Several studies in patients with diabetes or impaired glucose tolerance have shown magnesium to be of value. Magnesium supplementation, usually 400–500 milligrams per day, improves insulin response and action, glucose tolerance, and the fluidity of the red blood cell membrane. In addition, magnesium levels are usually low in diabetics and lowest in those with severe retinopathy. Diabetics complaining of fatigue appear to have higher magnesium requirements. An underlying magnesium deficiency can result in symptoms similar to those of chronic fatigue syndrome. Low red blood cell magnesium levels, a more accurate measure of magnesium status than routine blood analysis, have been found in many patients with chronic fatigue syndrome. Double-blind studies in people with chronic fatigue syndrome have shown that magnesium supplementation significantly improved energy levels, emotional state, and pain. These more recent studies support the results from clinical trials during 1960s on patients suffering from chronic fatigue. The earlier studies utilized oral magnesium and potassium aspartate and found that between 75 and 91% of the nearly 3,000 patients studied experienced relief of fatigue during treatment. In contrast, the number of patients responding to placebo was between 9 and 26%. The beneficial effect was usually noted after only 4 or 5 days but sometimes 10 days were required. Patients usually continued treatment for 4–6 weeks. The recommended daily allowance of magnesium for a pregnant woman is 350 mg of supplementation. That is the upper limit; however, if you are getting magnesium from foods or drinks or other sources, this is not added into your 350 mg total. This is the amount you should be taking in supplements, but if you are getting more than that in food, that is okay. You do not need to decrease the amount of supplement you take because you eat magnesium-rich foods.

Fibromyalgia is a recently recognized disorder regarded as a common cause of chronic muscular skeletal pain and fatigue. One study demonstrated that a daily supplement of 300–600 milligrams of magnesium malate resulted in tremendous improvement in the number of severity of tender points. Magnesium increases the solubility of calcium in the urine, thereby preventing kidney stone formation. Supplementing magnesium in the diet has demonstrated significant effect improving recurrences of kidney stones. However, when used in conjunction with bitamin B-6, an even greater effect is noted. In migraine and tension headaches there is considerable evidence that low magnesium levels trigger both migraine and tension headaches in individuals with low magnesium levels. Magnesium supplementation has been shown to produce excellent results in double-blind studies.

Magnesium needs increase during pregnancy as reflected in an increase in the recommended daily allowance from 280 milligrams for adults to 350 milligrams per day for pregnant women. Magnesium deficiency during pregnancy has been linked to preeclampsia, a severe condition of pregnancy associated with elevations in blood pressure, fluid retention and loss of protein in the urine, pre-term delivery, and fetal growth retardation. In contrast, supplementing the diet of pregnant women with additional oral magnesium has been shown to significantly decrease the incidence of these complications. Magnesium is frequently found in conjunction with calcium supplements but it can also be found alone. Caution: If you suffer from a serious kidney disorder or are on hemodialysis, do not take magnesium supplements unless directed to do so by a physician. People with severe heart disease or an arrhythmia also should not take magnesium or potassium unless under direct supervision of a physician.

In general, magnesium is very well tolerated, but there are some possible side effects. Magnesium supplementation can sometimes cause a looser stool, particularly with the use of magnesium sulfate, magnesium hydroxide, or magnesium chloride. There are many drugs that appear to adversely affect magnesium status. Most notable are many diuretics, antacids and ulcer medication, insulin, and digitalis. Magnesium supplements should not be taken within two hours of these drugs.

Many nutritional experts feel that the ideal intake for magnesium should be based on body weight; 6 milligrams per kilogram or 2.2 pounds of body weight. Therefore, for a 110-pound person, the recommendation would be 300 milligrams; for a 154-pound person, 420 milligrams; and for a 200-pound person, 540 milligrams. Usually overdosage results in diarrhea, and the magnesium is considered safe during pregnancy and lactation at the recommended dietary allowance of 350 milligrams daily.

Magnesium nutritional status can be influenced by a number of factors, but the easiest to correct is magnesium intake. Not all prenatal supplements used in the United States contain magnesium. Within the last few years, more include magnesium than previously. Magnesium is usually included in the form of magnesium oxide, which is 60% magnesium by weight. If magnesium is included in a prenatal supplement, it is normally added in amounts of 100 milligrams of elemental magnesium. There is no evidence concerning the bio-availability of magnesium contained in these supplements. Prenatal supplements do not provide enough magnesium to meet the recommended daily allowance because most dietary intakes are less than 300 milligrams. Additional magnesium supplementation for pregnant women is recommended. Usually in prenatal vitamins, when magnesium is present, it is found in levels between 25 and 200 milligrams. There is a wide variation in magnesium present in prenatal vitamins. Usually the ones in the health food store will contain amounts closer to the 200 milligram range. The prescription prenatal vitamins will be between 25 and 75 milligrams.

A paper on magnesium was presented at the Fourth International Symposium on Magnesium, July 23–28, 1985. The abstract mentions that the mean dietary magnesium intake of pregnant women is 35–58% of the recommended dietary allowance of 450 milligrams. Low-income women consumed 97–100 milligrams of magnesium per 1000 kilocalories, whereas women with higher incomes averaged 120 milligrams per 1000 kilocalories. Diets high in fat and sugar and low in whole grains, vegetables, and fruits have a lower magnesium density. Magnesium content of water can also make a significant contribution to magnesium intake.

There is a growing literature that provides evidence that a compromised magnesium nutritional status may be involved in several disorders that can occur during pregnancy. These include hypertension, vasospasm, coagulation defects, premature delivery, intrauterine growth retardation, and muscle cramping. Magnesium deficiency in general can be difficult to diagnose and correlate with clinical symptoms because about 50% of the total body magnesium is stored in the bones and only 1% of the remaining part is to be found in the extra-cellular compartment. One double-blind trial of 73 pregnant women found that three weeks of magnesium supplements significantly reduced leg cramps as compared to the placebo. This was in *The American Journal of Obstetrics and Gynecology*, 1995, Volume 173, pages 175–180.

Selenium

The trace marrow selenium functions primarily as a component of the antioxidant enzyme glutathione peroxidase, which works with vitamin E in preventing free radical damage to cell membranes. Low levels of selenium have been linked to a higher risk of cancer, cardiovascular disease, inflammatory diseases, and other conditions associated with increased free radical damage, including premature aging and cataract formation. Severe selenium deficiency is associated with Keshan Disease, which is a serious heart disorder that affects primarily children and women of childbearing age in some areas of China where selenium levels in the soil are very low. However, severe selenium deficiency states are extremely rare in North America. More common is a chronically low selenium intake that is associated with an increased risk for cancer, an increased risk of heart disease, and low immune function. Selenium levels have been shown to be low in patients with rheumatoid arthritis, eczema, and psoriasis. Clinical studies have not yet clearly demonstrated that selenium supplementation alone improves inflammatory conditions. For example, a study with selenium alone showed no benefit for rheumatoid arthritis. However, one clinical study of rheumatoid arthritis patients indicated that selenium combined with vitamin E did provide some benefit. Supplementing the diet with 50–200 micrograms of selenium and 200–400 international units of vitamin E appears to be appropriate in inflammatory conditions due to an increased need, the low selenium levels typically seen in inflammatory conditions (in nonpregnant patients), and selenium and vitamin E's synergistic effects of antioxidants.

There is substantial evidence that selenium is essential for proper fetal growth and development. Selenium requirements appear to be increased during pregnancy as selenium concentrations in the blood tend to be lower during pregnancy, particularly during the later stages. Selenium levels tend to be very low in low-birth-weight babies. Do not take selenium at levels greater than those recommended because significant toxicity can occur at higher intake levels. Do not exceed 60 micrograms daily of supplemental selenium in pregnancy.

Possible side effects. The human body requires just a small amount of selenium. Dosages as low as 900 micrograms per day over prolonged periods of time can produce signs of selenium toxicity in some people. Signs and symptoms related to chronic toxicity include depression, nervousness, emotional instability, nausea and vomiting, a garlic odor of the breath and sweat, and in extreme cases also of hair and fingernails.

Selenium absorption is adversely affected by high dosages of vitamin C and by high intakes of other trace minerals, particularly zinc. Selenium works closely with vitamin E and antioxidant mechanisms. Although there is no specific recommended daily allowance for selenium, for non-pregnant adults a daily intake of 50–200 micrograms is often recommended. Selenium supplementation is suitable during pregnancy and lactation at recommended levels. Selenium may be missing from your prenatal vitamin.

Zinc

Zinc is a trace mineral that is found in virtually every cell in the body and is a component in more than 200 enzymes. Low zinc levels affect virtually every system of the body. Zinc is also required for proper action of many hormones, including insulin, growth hormones, and sex hormones. Zinc is especially important to proper immune function, wound healing, sensory functions, sexual function, and skin health.

Severe zinc deficiency is very rare in developed countries, it is believed that many individuals in the United States have marginal zinc deficiency. Especially in the elderly population, the zinc deficiency can be caused by decreased intake and/or utilization. Dietary surveys indicate that average zinc intakes range from only 47% to 67% of the recommended daily allowance. Marginal zinc deficiency may be reflected by an increased susceptibility to infection, poor wound healing, a decreased sense of taste or smell, and a number of minor skin disorders including acne, eczema, and psoriasis. Other physical findings that often correlate with low zinc status include decreased ability to see at night or with poor lighting, growth retardation, testicular atrophy, mouth ulcers, a white coating on the tongue, and marked halitosis.

For the common cold, zinc possesses some indirect antiviral activity. The use of zinc supplementation, particularly in the form of a lozenge, appears to be of value during a cold; however, out of eight double-blind studies, four found zinc lozenges to be effective while the other four reported no difference between zinc and placebo therapy. This inconsistency is thought to be due to an ineffective lozenge formulation in the negative studies. It appears that in order for zinc to be effective it must be ionized in the saliva.

Low zinc levels are linked to premature births, low birth weight, growth retardation, and preeclampsia, a serious condition of pregnancy associated with elevations in blood pressure, fluid retention, and loss of protein in the urine. Studies of zinc supplementation in pregnancy have shown that infants born to the zinc-supplemented mothers had greater body weight and head circumference compared to the placebo group. Zinc-supplemented mothers also had fewer complications of pregnancy. Do not take more than the recommended amounts, especially if pregnant or lactating. If taken on an empty stomach, zinc supplementation can result in gastrointestinal upset and nausea. Zinc supplements should be taken separately from high-fiber foods for best absorption. High doses of calcium or iron can adversely affect zinc absorption. When using zinc-containing lozenges for the relief of a sore throat or common cold, do not eat or drink citrus fruits or juices one-half hour before or after. The citric acid will negate the effect of zinc. The usual dosage range for zinc supplementation for general health support during pregnancy or lactation is 15–20 milligrams.

When zinc supplementation is being used to address specific health concerns, the dosage range for women is between 20 and 30 milligrams. For the common cold, use lozenges that supply 15–25 milligrams of elemental zinc and dissolve them in the mouth without chewing every two waking hours. After an initial double dose, continue for only up to seven days because high doses of zinc can actually impair immune function. A daily intake of greater than 150 milligrams of zinc for longer than one week cannot be recommended. Acute toxicity is quite rare as the ingestion of amounts large enough to cause toxicity symptoms will usually provoke vomiting. The upper limit of zinc in pregnancy is 40 milligrams daily. Most prenatal vitamins available by prescription will have between 15 and 25 milligrams. The recommended daily allowance of zinc for pregnancy women is 15, for lactating women it's 19.

Essential Fatty Acids

Some experts estimate that as much as 80% of the United States population consumes an insufficient quantity of essential fatty acids. This dietary insufficiency presents a serious health threat to Americans. Essential fatty acids are important for the regulation of a host of bodily functions including inflammation, pain and swelling, blood pressure, heart function, gastrointestinal function and secretions, kidney function and fluid balance, blood clotting and platelet aggregation, allergic responses, nerve transmission and steroid production, and hormone synthesis. The signs and symptoms of essential fatty acid deficiency may be either quite obvious or somewhat hard to detect. Most formulas for feeding newborns have been fortified with essential fatty acids, and now many prescription prenatal vitamins include an additional fatty acid supplement in the packaging.

Essential fatty acids have desirable affects on many disorders. They improve the skin and hair, reduce blood pressure, aide in the prevention of arthritis, lower cholesterol and triglyceride levels, and reduce the risk of blood clot formation. They are beneficial for candidiasis, cardiovascular disease, eczema, and psoriasis. Found in high concentrations in the brain, essential fatty acids aid in the transmission of nerve impulses and are needed for the normal development and functioning of the brain. A deficiency of essential fatty acids can lead to an inability to learn and recall information.

There are two basic categories of essential fatty acids, designated omega-3 and omega-6, based on their chemical structures. Omega-3 fatty acids are found in fresh deepwater fish, fish oil, and certain vegetable oils, among them canola oil, flaxseed oil, and walnut oil. Omega-6 fatty acids, which include linoleic and gamma linoleic acids, are found primarily in raw nuts, seeds and legumes, and in unsaturated vegetable oils, such as borage oil, grape seed oil, primrose oil, and sesame oil. Fish oils are useful in allergies, eczema, and asthma. Omega-3 fatty acids are important mediators of allergy and inflammation. Some double-blind studies indicate that fish oil supplementation may help reduce inflammation and allergic reactions in eczema, asthma, and other allergic disorders. There is also considerable evidence from more than 30 double-blind studies that fish oil supplementation reduces blood triglyceride levels, especially in patients with severe elevations. Most but not all of these double-blind studies have also shown that fish oils lower blood cholesterol levels. The typical decrease in triglyceride levels with fish oil supplementation is 20–50%. Results are usually apparent within the first month. In double-blind studies, patients with psoriasis have been successfully treated with fish oil.

Insufficiency of omega-3 oils in the diet has been linked to depression, manic-depression, and schizophrenia. Preliminary evidence indicates that fish oil supplementation may help improve brain function, mood, and behavior in people suffering from these psychological disorders. Autoimmune diseases, such as rheumatoid arthritis, lupus, and multiple sclerosis are characterized by the immune system actually attacking the body's own tissue. The result is tremendous inflammation and tissue destruction in the area being attacked. There is mounting evidence that fish oil supplementation may beneficially influence the course of treatment in patients with these autoimmune diseases. Fish oil supplements are available primarily in soft gelatin capsules. Be sure that the product is fish oil, not fish liver oil. This distinction is important, especially in pregnant women, because fish liver oil contains fat-soluble vitamins A and D, which if taken in excessive amounts have the potential to cause toxicity.

Fish oil is generally safe in pregnancy. Individuals with diabetes must monitor blood sugar levels closely if electing to use fish oil supplements. Elevations in blood sugar and cholesterol levels have occurred in some diabetics taking fish oil. The most common side effect with fish oil supplementation is mild gastrointestinal upset. Some people may burp up a fishy smell. And because fish oil supplementation may reduce platelet stickiness, it may also increase the risk of bleeding in patients taking coumadin and aspirin.

Flaxseed Oil

Flaxseed oil is unique because it contains two essential fatty acids, alpha linoleic acid an omega-6 fatty acid, in high amounts. Increasing the intake of omega-3 fatty acids from either fish oil supplements or flaxseed oil can lower blood pressure. Although the fish oils typically have a more pronounced effect than flaxseed oil, one study indicated that along with reducing the intake of saturated fat, one tablespoon per day of flaxseed oil dropped both the systolic and diastolic blood pressure readings by up to nine millimeters of mercury. Flaxseed oil is available in liquid form in bottles and soft gelatin capsules. This is considered safe in pregnancy and lactation.

Inositol

Inositol is an unofficial member of the B vitamin group that functions as a primary component of cell membranes. However, inositol has not been shown to be essential in the human diet. Supplementation has been shown to exert some beneficial effects in cases of depression, panic disorder, and diabetes. Inositol is required for the proper action of several neurotransmitters including serotonin and acetylcholine. It is currently thought that a reduction of brain inositol levels may induce depression because inositol levels in the cerebral spinal fluid have been shown to be low with depression. In double-blind studies, inositol at a dosage of 12 grams per day has demonstrated therapeutic results. It shows a reduction in score on the Hamilton Depression Scale similar to those tricyclic antidepressant drugs but without the side effects. Because of the effect of inositol on depression, a double-blind study was designed to test inositol's effectiveness on panic disorder. The frequency and severity of panic attacks declined significantly, more after inositol at 12 grams per day than after placebo administration. Further studies are needed to document this effect.

Inositol is showing some promise in diabetic neuropathy, a nerve disease caused by diabetes. There are no known possible side effects, no known drug interactions, no known effects of overdosage, and it is considered safe during pregnancy and lactation. Most prescription prenatal vitamins do not include this but it can be found in a prenatal vitamins in health food stores. If it were being recommended for depression or panic attacks, one would have to buy an extra supplement over-the-counter because 12 grams is recommended for these disorders.

Lactate

Lactate contains the enzyme lactase, which is necessary for digesting the sugar lactose from diary products. The enzyme is derived from a yeast. Deficiency in the enzyme lactase is common worldwide. Lactate is available in caplets or a liquid form and is considered safe in pregnancy and lactation at the doses that are recommended on the product.

Iodine

Iodine is an essential mineral needed for proper thyroid function, and a maternal iodine deficiency can cause significant irreversible mental retardation in the fetus. Iodine deficiency constitutes one of the most common preventable causes of mental deficiency in the world today. The American diet is abundant in salt, and an iodine deficiency in this country is rare. I have not instructed anyone to purchase a separate iodine supplement for the conditions I have described in this book.

Lactobacillus acidophilus

Lactobacillus acidophilus are friendly bacteria valued for their health-promoting properties. Lactobacilli are key components of proper intestinal aura. Lactobacilli produce a variety of factors that inhibit or antagonize other bacteria. Lactobacillus supplementation has shown good results in preventing and treating antibiotic-induced diarrhea. Antibiotics often cause diarrhea by altering the type of bacteria in the colon or by promoting the overgrowth of candida albicans. It appears that when antibiotics are necessary it is important to supplement with lactobacilli. Lactobacillus acidophilus has been shown to retard the growth of candida albicans, which is the major yeast involved in vaginal yeast infections. Clinical studies have suggested that the introduction of lactobacilli to the vagina can assist in clearing of yeast infections and preventing their recurrent infections as well as preventing bacterial vaginosis. Lactobacillus is generally regarded as safe for use during pregnancy and lactation; overdosage generally results in excessive flatulence and possibly diarrhea.

Liver Extracts

Liver extracts are used for iron-deficiency anemia and hepatitis. Extracts of beef liver are a rich, natural source of many vitamins and minerals including iron. Liver extracts provide the most absorbable form of iron, heme iron, and other nutrients critical in building blood, including vitamin B-12 and folic acid. Liver extracts can contain as much as 3–4 milligrams of heme iron per gram. In addition to its use as a source of iron, liver extracts are used to support liver function and boost energy levels. Liver extracts are available as nutritional supplements in capsules and tablets. Liver extracts should not be used in patients suffering from an iron storage disorder such has hemochromatosis. There are no known possible side effects. There are no known drug interactions. There are no known food and nutrient interactions. For usual dosage, instructions on the label should be followed. There is no known overdosage issue and it is considered safe during pregnancy and lactation.

SAMe

SAMe, stands for S-adenosylmethionine. SAMe is formed in the body by combining the essential amino acid, methionine, to adenosine-triphosphate, ATP. It is involved in more than 40 biochemical reactions in the body. It functions closely with folic acid and vitamin B-12 in methylation reactions. Currently the main uses of SAMe are in the treatment of depression, fibromyalgia, liver disorders, migraine headaches, and osteoarthritis. Based on results from a number of clinical studies, it appears that SAMe is the perhaps the most effective natural anti-depressant. In fact, in these studies SAMe has demonstrated better results that conventional anti-depressant drugs and fewer side effects. In addition to generalized depression, SAMe has produced significant effects in relieving postpartum depression and to reduce the anxiety and depression associated with drug detoxification and rehabilitation. SAMe's anti-depressant effects are related to its ability to increase levels of important brain chemicals such as serotonin, dopamine, and phosphatidylserine. SAMe also leads to improved binding of serotonin and dopamine to their receptor sites. SAMe has been shown to be quite beneficial in several other disorders, including cirrhosis. Clinical studies have shown that SAMe is quite useful in protecting the liver from damage and improving liver function in conditions associated with estrogen excess, namely oral contraceptive use, pregnancy, and premenstrual syndrome.

Fibromyalgia is a recently recognized disorder regarded as a common cause of chronic musculoskeletal pain and fatigue. SAMe has been shown in at least four clinical studies to produce excellent benefits in patients suffering from fibromyalgia. Improvements were indicated by a significant reduction in the number of trigger points and painful areas as well as improvements in mood. SAMe has also been shown to be a benefit in the treatment of migraine headaches. The benefit arises gradually and long-term treatment is required for therapeutic effectiveness. SAMe is available in capsules and tablets. It has been available in commercially in Europe since 1975 and was introduced in the United States in 1998. Individuals with bipolar disorder should not take SAMe unless under strict medical supervision because SAMe's antidepressant activity may lead to the manic phase in these individuals. No side effects have been reported with oral SAMe other than occasional nausea and gastrointestinal disturbances. There are no known drug, food or nutrient interactions. SAMe is usually recommended at a dosage of 200–400 milligrams, twice per day. There are no known effects of overdosage and it is considered safe in pregnancy and lactation.

Other Botanicals

Bilberry

Bilberry, also known as the European Blueberry, has an active compound known as anthocyanidin. It has been shown to be a potent antioxidant that improves the integrity and function of small blood vessels. Bilberry extracts are thought to be helpful in varicose veins because of their ability to strengthen the vein wall and improve vein function. Clinical studies have shown that bilberry extracts reduce swelling; feelings of heaviness; a pins-and-needles sensation; pain; and skin changes in patients with varicose veins. Bilberry extracts are available in capsules and tablets. There are no cautions and warnings or side effects for bilberry extracts that have been reported. Bilberry extracts have no known toxic effects and are considered safe during pregnancy and lactation.

Cranberry

Cranberry juice and cranberry extracts have shown benefit in preventing and treating urinary tract infections in several double-blind studies. For example, in one study of 153 women with active urinary tract infections, 16 fluid ounces of Ocean Spray Cranberry drink per day produced beneficial effects in 73% of the subjects. When the cranberry juice was withdrawn, 61% of the women experienced a recurrence of their bladder infection. Many believe that the action of cranberry juice is due to acidifying the urine into the antibacterial effects of hippuric acid, a component of cranberries. However, in order to acidify the urine, at least one quart of cranberry juice would have to be consumed at one sitting and even then the concentration of hippuric acid in the urine as a result of drinking cranberry juice is insufficient to inhibit bacteria. Dehydrated cranberry juice and cranberry extracts are available in capsules and tablets. Recent studies have shown that components of cranberry juice reduce the ability of bacteria such as *E-coli* to adhere to the lining of the bladder and urethra. In order for bacteria to infect, they must first adhere to the mucosal lining. By interfering with adherence, cranberry juice or extracts greatly reduce the likelihood of infection and allow the body to marshal its own defenses. One should consult a physician, especially if one is pregnant, if you have symptoms suggestive of a bladder infection, such as pain or burning on urination, increased urinary frequency, or cloudy, foul-smelling dark urine. But in people who have a history of a urinary tract infection or have them often and would like to prevent or delay a recurrence, I recommend cranberry juice or a cranberry supplement daily. There are no known possible side effects, no known drug interactions, no known food and nutrient interactions, and no known overdosage effects. It is considered safe during pregnancy and lactation.

Echinacea

Echinacea can be used for the common cold, and I have recommended it to my patients for this purpose. It is generally safe in pregnancy. Allergic reactions, however, have been reported in people who are allergic to ragweed. The majority of studies have suggested that Echinacea displays an ability to reduce the duration and severity of cold symptoms. The evidence in prevention of the common cold is inconclusive.

Using the herb Echinacea during pregnancy does not increase the risk of birth defects in babies, according to work by researchers at Toronto's Hospital for Children. Echinacea, a supplement thought to stimulate the immune system, is one of the most popular herbal medicines on the North American market. It is used primarily for the prevention and treatment of upper respiratory infections; however, little data has been available to show its safety in pregnant women. In the study published in the November 13, 2000 issue of *The Archives of Internal Medicine*, researchers followed up on about 200 women who had contacted the Motherisk Program regarding the use of Echinacea during pregnancy. Motherisk provides information and guidance on the potential effects of drugs, disease, and other factors on the developing fetus or infant. Some of the women had taken the supplement knowing that they were pregnant, whereas others used it while unaware of being pregnant. This group was compared to another group of about 200 pregnant women who did not use Echinacea. The researchers compared the rates of live births, miscarriages, and major and minor birth defects between the two groups and found no statistical differences between them.

Elderberry

Elderberry is also a remedy for the common cold. It has been a popular flu and common cold remedy since the time of the Romans. Recent research has demonstrated that elderberry juice not only stimulates the immune system but also directly inhibits the influenza virus. In clinical trials, patients with influenza who took elderberry juice syrup reported faster termination of symptoms. Twenty percent reported significant improvement within 24 hours; 70% felt better by 48 hours; and 90% claimed a complete cure after three days. Patients receiving the placebo required six days for recovery. Elderberry extracts and syrups are available in liquid form, tablets, and capsules. Elderberry flowers and dried berries are also available in bulk to make tea. There are no known cautions and warnings, no known possible side effects, no drug interactions, no food and nutrient interactions, no overdosage issues, and it is generally considered safe during pregnancy and lactation.

Ginger

Another herb that I counsel my pregnant patients to use is ginger. It is effective for nausea and vomiting during pregnancy and also motion sickness. Nausea and vomiting is not necessarily related to first trimester morning sickness, and migraine headaches. There have been a few case reports of ginger's being helpful in migraine headaches, but this application has not been reported by a formal clinical trial. Ginger was first shown to be effective in treating morning sickness in a 1982 journal article. Since this time there have been several follow-up studies showing positive effects. Unlike anti-motion sickness drugs that act primarily on the brain and inner ear, ginger appears to exert its effects primarily by partially inhibiting the excessive stomach mobility characteristic of motion sickness.

Although the overall effectiveness of ginger in motion has yet to be determined, it is certainly a safe recommendation with some evidence of effectiveness.

Ginger also appears somewhat useful in the treatment of drug-induced and post-operative nausea and vomiting. In one study for nausea and vomiting during pregnancy, 250 milligrams of dried ginger root powder administered four times per day brought about a significant reduction in both the severity of the nausea and the number of attacks of vomiting in 19 out of 27 cases studies during early pregnancy, which is defined as less than 20 weeks. These preliminary clinical results along with ginger's safety and the relatively small dose required support the use of ginger to treat nausea and vomiting in pregnancy. Most studies have used powdered ginger root but fresh ginger is also thought to be effective. There are no cautions or warnings, no signs of overdosage, and it is considered safe during pregnancy and lactation. Possible side effects occur at dosages of 6000 milligrams or more; powdered, dried ginger has been shown to irritate the lining of the stomach. For nausea and vomiting of pregnancy, 1000 milligrams per day is usually sufficient.

Peppermint

The most popular medicinal uses of peppermint and peppermint oil are for the treatment of the common cold and irritable bowel syndrome. Peppermint oil is also used extensively in antacid products, irritants, laxatives, and mouthwash both for its flavor and for its therapeutic effects. Menthol and peppermint oil are often components of cough and throat lozenges as well as ointments, salves, and inhalants. Benefits of these products have not been proven in clinical studies but they are generally regarded as effective. Their popularity appears to be based on their ability to ease breathing difficulties during the common cold. Peppermint tea and peppermint oil have long been used to calm intestinal spasms and reduce excessive flatulence. There is evidence to support this historical use. Peppermint oil has been shown in several clinical studies to be quite helpful in the treatment of irritable bowel syndrome. This syndrome is characterized by a combination of any of the following symptoms: abdominal pain and distension and more frequent bowel movements with pain. Overdosage with peppermint tea has not been reported;

however, overdosage is possible with peppermint oil. For pregnant women, I recommend that only the peppermint tea be used.

Garlic

Garlic should not be taken during pregnancy since it has abortifacient properties. It should also be avoided during lactation because it has been shown to enter breast milk, altering the odor of the milk and affecting the suckling behavior of the infant. This is taken from *The Complimentary Medicines Summary for Garlic Supplements* produced December 13, 2002.

Choline

Choline works together with folic acid, ditamin B12, S-adenosylmethionine, and vitamin B6, and it helps the body conserve carnitine and folic acid. It can be manufactured by the body. Without choline, fats become trapped in the liver, where they block metabolism. I have not seen any studies that relate this substance to weight gain in pregnancy, but this would be an interesting thing to study. It is required for the export of fat in the liver. I have seen it in a couple of prenatal vitamins in the amount of 5–10 mg. Choline at high dosages (20 mg) will produce a fishy odor.

Supplements Taken by Disease

Anxiety

Anxiety can range from feeling hyper-aware and uneasy, and startling easily all the way to full-blown panic attacks. Headache and chronic fatigue are common among people with chronic anxiety. If you are on medications for anxiety, please consult your physician before you discontinue them. If you are on benzodiazapines, such as Valium, Librium, or Xanax, consult with your obstetrician immediately, as they are not recommended in pregnancy.

Supplements that are helpful:

- Vitamin C: 500–2000 milligrams
- B-Complex 50
- Calcium and magnesium supplements: Calcium is a natural tranquilizer, and magnesium helps to relieve anxiety, tension, muscle spasms, and tics. It is best taken in combination with calcium.
- Inositol: Can be taken up to 12 grams daily.
- SAMe: Can be taken up to 400 milligrams, twice daily. It should not be taken if you have manic depressive disorder or take prescription antidepressants.
- Fish oil
- Pantothenic acid: 100–500 milligrams
- Gotu kola: An herb that has been given to pregnant women in Italy; 260 milligrams, three times per day
- Chamomile tea: Can promote relaxation, but should be avoided if you are allergic to ragweed

A body under stress is more vulnerable to free-radical damage. Most prenatal vitamins, and multivitamins in general, contain the recommended daily allowance of 30 international units of vitamin E. I recommend supplementing with 200–400 international units of vitamin E. These supplements are meant to be taken in addition to your multivitamin.

Anemia

Millions of Americans suffer from anemia, which is a reduction either in the number of red blood cells or the amount of hemoglobin in the blood. This results in a decrease in the amount of oxygen that the blood is able to carry. Before you start treating yourself for anemia, make sure your doctor recommends that you take medicine for anemia. The most common cause of anemia is iron deficiency; however, a person can have a B-12 or folic acid deficiency that is causing anemia. Also, it is important to rule out underlying diseases because sometimes anemia, in and of itself, might not be a disease but a symptom of various other diseases, such as arthritis, infection, or cancer. It is also important to rule out blood loss as a reason for the anemia. For instance, an ulcer or some other hidden bleeding could be causing the anemia. So before supplementing yourself, make sure that you have spoken to your doctor to rule out more serious problems.

Of course, iron is recommended for iron deficiency anemia. Ferrous sulfate is my least favorite kind, simply because patients often complain of it's symptoms, such as gas, bloating, constipation, and nausea, but it is inexpensive and easy to obtain without a prescription. Ferrous fumarate and Ferrous gluconate are better tolerated. Carbonyl iron, which is found in the prenatal vitamin supplements occasionally, is a form that is easier to tolerate. It is a good idea to take iron with vitamin C and folic acid. Even if a patient does not have folic acid deficiency, taking vitamin C with folic acid along with the iron can help to improve the anemia faster. Low zinc levels may worsen iron deficiency anemia. Up to 40 milligrams is safe in pregnancy. Vitamin C does enhance the absorption of iron, so your iron supplement should be taken with orange juice or a vitamin C supplement. They come in convenient 500-milligram tablets.

Blackstrap molasses can be taken for anemia if a person doesn't like taking pills are finds the aforementioned forms of iron difficult to tolerate. One tablespoon twice a day can be taken. It can be added to milk for a different taste. It contains iron and essential B vitamins. You can take this in addition to the prenatal vitamin.

Vitamin B-complex can be taken. B vitamins work best when taken together.

Raw liver extract is also a good way to increase the iron content of blood. It contains all the elements needed for red blood cell production. Use liver from organically raised beef. Five hundred milligrams twice a day is the usual dosage.

Allergies (Supplements to be taken to improve allergy symptoms)

Here, I am specifically referring to seasonal allergies. That is the type you would be taking Allegra, Zyrtec, or Claritin for. I live in Houston and I have countless patients who find these medicines beneficial but hesitate to take them while pregnant. An allergy is an inappropriate response by the body's immune system to a substance that is not normally harmful. Typical allergic responses are fever, congestion, coughing, wheezing, itching, shortness of breath, headache, fatigue, and hives and other skin rashes. Almost any substance can cause an allergic reaction in someone, somewhere in the world but the most common allergens are pollen, dust, certain metals, some cosmetics, lanolin, dust mites, animal hair, insect venom, some common drugs, some food additives such as benzylic acid and sulphur dioxide, animal dander, and chemicals found in soap, washing powder, cleaning supplies, and many other chemicals. Many people are allergic to mold.

- Vitamin C with bioflavinoids, 500–1000 mg, once or twice a day
- Pantothenic acid, 100–300 mg per day
- Vitamin B-complex
- Zinc, 20 mg per day
- Selenium, 60 micrograms per day
- Acidophilus, a powerful immune enhancer with digestive enzymes for improved digestion
- Quercetin, 500 mg twice daily, increases immunity and decreases reactions to certain foods, pollens, and other allergens
- Bromelain, 100 mg twice daily, enhances absorption of quercetin and reduces inflammation

I also recommend that a person purchase an air filter to clean pollen, mold, and dust in one's home and office.

<u>Asthma</u>

Asthma is recurring attacks of breathlessness, usually accompanied by wheezing or mild coughing. Although asthma frequently begins before the age of five, it can develop at any age. More than 10 million Americans have asthma. It is difficult to cure but can be controlled by avoiding triggers. Symptoms include trouble breathing, a tight feeling in the chest, and coughing and wheezing. Triggers may be pollen, house dust, animal fur or dander, smoking or exposure to secondhand tobacco smoke, exercise, stress, or anxiety. Some people can have food allergies that trigger their asthma, such as to cow's milk, shellfish, tomatoes, chocolate, fish, nuts, and food colorings, especially yellow dye number 5. If you are on asthma medications, please review them with your obstetrician. All of the asthma treatments that are safe in pregnancy are compatible with adding nutritional supplementation. One does not need to discontinue her asthma medications and should not do so unless under the advice of a doctor.

Regular use of a high-potency, multivitamin mineral supplement can reduce the number and severity of asthma attacks.

Taking up to 100 mg of vitamin B-6 in divided doses can decrease the number and severity asthma attacks.

Magnesium, up to the maximum of 350 mg per day, can also be taken, and in divided doses.

Vitamin C, up to 2000 mg per day in divided doses, can be taken. Taking the last dose before bed seems to decrease or lessen severity of attacks at 4 a.m.

Folic acid should also be taken. It is already in your multivitamin supplement, and if you are already taking vitamin B-6, you could get B-complex supplement so that the B-6 and the folic acid would both be present.

Essential fatty acids are useful for production of antiinflammatory prostaglandins.

Pantothenic is an antistress vitamin that can help reduce the triggers of asthma. This could be in the B-complex vitamin with the B-6 and folic acid that I've already recommended.

Beta carotene is in most prenatal vitamins, but if you do not already have beta carotene, you could take it up to 10,000 daily or vitamin A up to 5000 international units daily.

Selenium is a powerful destroyer of free radicals created from air pollutants; 60 mcg/day is a good dose in pregnancy.

Carpal Tunnel Syndrome

Carpal tunnel syndrome is a disorder that occurs from pressure on the median nerve as it passes through the carpal tunnel, a narrow, hollow area in the wrist. Surgery for carpal tunnel is a very common procedure in the United States. However, during pregnancy it is not that common for the procedure to be done, and if the procedure is secondary to the fluid gain of pregnancy, it usually resolves postpartum without surgical intervention. It is very likely to occur during the last trimester of pregnancy after weight and fluid gain are at their peak. Symptoms include numbness, tingling, and pain in the thumb, index, and middle fingers, wrist, or palm that often worsens at night. Other symptoms include stiffness of the wrist in the morning, cramping of the hand, inability to make a fist, weakness in the thumb, a feeling of burning in the finger, and a tendency to drop things. The causes of carpal tunnel syndrome are repetitive actions that keep the wrist flexed up or down, sleeping in this position, and wrist injury. People especially at risk are data-processors, cashiers, assembly-line workers, knitters and needle workers, and those who drive for hours at a time. The syndrome affects one out of every 10 Americans who work on computer terminals. Vitamin B-6 deficiency can cause carpal tunnel syndrome. For pregnancy, the only supplement I recommend for this syndrome is vitamin B-6. Your prenatal vitamin will have vitamin B-6 in it, most likely; however, an extra supplement is warranted. I recommend up to the 100 milligrams, which is the upper safe limit in pregnancy. Other things that help carpal tunnel syndrome are wrist splints placed on at night to immobilize the wrist and give the nerve relief from compression. Check your thyroid function and medication. Low thyroid and certain medications can cause carpal tunnel symptoms. Get up from your computer at least once every hour and stretch. Yoga arm postures, such as putting hands together in the prayer or greeting position, for several minutes twice a day may help prevent and heal carpal tunnel syndrome. At the first sign of symptoms, start increasing your dosage of vitamin B-6. Of course, at that point it's too late to prevent it but it is hoped that the progression will not be as great and you won't lose the use of your hands. If you have experienced this condition in a prior pregnancy, I recommend starting the extra vitamin B-6 early in the pregnancy. If you were taking vitamin B-6 in early pregnancy secondary to morning sickness, then continue it throughout the pregnancy and maybe doing so will decrease the likelihood that you will develop carpal tunnel syndrome again.

The increased frequency of carpal tunnel syndrome since 1950 parallels the increased presence of compounds that interfere with vitamin b-6 in the body. Particularly incriminating is tartrazine, which is yellow dye number five. Yellow dye number five is added to almost every packaged food. In the United Sates the average daily per capita consumption of certified dyes is 15 milligrams, of which 85% is tartrazine. Elimination of food dyes from the diet may alleviate carpal tunnel syndrome. The two natural medicines in which supplementation is found to be of benefit is vitamin B-6 and bromelain, which is found in pineapple.

Celiac Disease

Celiac disease, also called celiac sprue, is a chronic digestive disorder that is caused by a hereditary intolerance to gluten. Gluten is a component of wheat, rye, oats, barley, and related grain derivatives. The cause of celiac disease is unknown, although it is known mostly to affect Caucasians of European descent. When a person with celiac disease consumes gluten, damage to the small intestine results. It is believed that the body responds to gluten as though it were an antigen and launches an immune system attack when the gluten is absorbed by the intestine. This in turn causes the lining of the small intestine to swell. Malabsorption subsequently becomes a serious problem, and the loss of vitamins, minerals, and calories results in malnutrition despite an adequate diet. Diarrhea compounds the problem. Because celiac disease impairs digestion, food allergies may also appear. Celiac disease affects both adults and children and can appear at any age. It often appears when a child is first introduced to cereal foods at or around three months of age. In others, the disease can be triggered by emotional stress or physical trauma such as a surgery or pregnancy. The first signs are usually diarrhea, weight loss, and nutritional deficiencies. The prevalence is approximately one of 500 persons in the United States. There is no known cure for celiac disease, but it can be controlled by lifelong adherence to a gluten-free diet. Supplements are as follows:

- Essential fatty acids: Needed for the villi in the intestines.
- A multivitamin: Make sure that it is wheat- and yeast-free.
- B-12 and folic acid: Can be found in a B-complex supplement. Sometimes it is necessary for these to be in the injectable form, secondary to the fact that most B vitamins are absorbed in the gut and the gut is malfunctioning during exacerbations of the disease. If it is taken orally, be sure that it is a wheat- and yeast-free product.

Magnesium deficiency is common in people with Celiac disease. In pregnancy, the upper limit that is acceptable is 350 milligrams daily. A magnesium plus calcium supplement are also good in pregnancy. A multivitamin is important, such as a prenatal vitamin, but vitamin E should be supplemented up to 400 international units daily. Fat-soluble vitamins are not well-dissolved in this disorder, so it is good to use additional supplementation beyond what is found in a multivitamin. Vitamin C should be given for the immune system. The maximum in pregnancy is 2000 milligrams per day. Psyllium fiber is also good to cleanse the colon.

Gluten-free products are available at health food stores. This is another condition in which blackstrap molasses is useful as it is high in iron and the B vitamins. It may be necessary to remove milk and milk products from the diet because of a secondary lactase deficiency. If milk does have to be consumed, Lactaid is safe in pregnancy. This is an over-the-counter supplement that helps to digest the enzyme lactose, which is the enzyme that people with lactose deficiency are missing.

Cervical Dysplasia

Cervical dysplasia is an abnormal condition of the cells of the cervix. It can also be known as an abnormal pap smear. It is generally regarded as a precancerous lesion and has risk factors similar to those of cervical cancer. It is quite probable that many abnormal pap smears reflect folate deficiency rather than true dysplasia, especially in women who are pregnant or are taking oral contraceptives, because estrogens antagonize folic acid. The human papillomavirus (HPV) exposure has been linked to the development of dysplasia, although many people with HPV never develop cervical cancer. Risk factors include: sex before age eighteen, multiple sexual partners, and smoking.

Folic acid supplementation, up to 10 mg/day, has resulted in improvement or normalization of pap smears in patients with cervical dysplasia in clinical studies. At this time, the upper limit of folic acid in pregnancy is 1 milligram. I do not recommend that a patient who is pregnant take that particular amount of folic acid, which is 10 times the amount in a prescription vitamin; however I would have that patient ensure that she is taking the maximum amount possible.

I generally recommend that my patients take increased amounts of antioxidants:

- Vitamin C: Up to 2000 milligrams is safe in pregnancy.
- Vitamin E, 400–800 international units, and folic acid: These have been studied and thought to improve abnormal pap smears.
- Beta carotene: 10,000 international units per day.

Common Cold

The common cold is an infection of the upper respiratory tract caused by a virus. There are more than 200 viruses that can cause the common cold, but the most common ones are rhinoviruses. The well-known symptoms include head congestion, nasal congestion, sore throat, coughing, headache, sneezing, and watery eyes. Most colds clear up on their own in a week to 10 days but occasionally a cold can lead to a more serious illness such as bronchitis, middle ear infection, or sinus infection. Please contact your physician if you have a fever greater than 102 before using any over-the-counter remedies.

For a sore throat, zinc and vitamin C lozenges are soothing. Vitamin C can also be taken in dosages up to 2000 mg daily. Make sure that your zinc total does not exceed 40 mg daily.

Make sure you are taking your prenatal vitamins.

Echinacea is also safe in pregnancy and can be taken for a cold.

Slippery elm is also something that is soothing on the throat and that has been used in pregnancy without consequence, although it has not been studied specifically for pregnancy. The slippery elm tree is native to North America. The inner bark of the tree is the source of a mucilage that historically have been used to soothe internal membranes irritated by the common cold, cough, ulcers, or inflammatory bowel disease such as Crohn's Disease and ulcerative colitis, but there have been no clinical studies documenting its effect. The FDA does allow products containing slippery elm to claim that they are of value in soothing a sore throat. Slippery elm is available as a tea and in capsules and tablets including chewable tablets and as throat lozenges. There are no known side effects. Slippery elm may interfere with the absorption of drugs, so take any medication at least 45 minutes before or after using slippery elm. It has no food or nutrient interactions, so it is something that can also be used if one has a sore throat in addition to one's cold. For sore throat, a mixture of raw honey and lemon juice to coat and soothe can be used. One can sip a tea made from chamomile to keep the throat lubricated. One can gargle with chlorophyl liquid in a glass of warm water or sea salt in a glass of warm water every few hours. If you smoke, stop. Smoking is a major cause of sore throats. Vitamin C is available in liquid form, or one could dissolve vitamin C powder in water or juice; this would be good to sip to allow it to soothe your sore throat.

Constipation

Constipation is difficulty in passing stools or the infrequent passage of hard, dry stools as a result of food moving slowly through the large intestine. Most people experience constipation from time to time, but usually lifestyle changes and better eating habits can help relieve the symptoms and prevent recurrences. The most common cause of constipation is a low-fiber diet. Other common causes include inadequate fluid intake, lack of physical activities, and various medications. Even the iron in your prenatal vitamins and antacids can be the most common culprits in pregnant women. Low thyroid function and irritable bowel syndrome are also medical problems that can contribute to this. The first thing I tell my pregnant patients to do when they complain of constipation is to increase their water intake. Not carbonated drinks, not milk, not juice, only water. Also, I recommend a high-fiber diet. One can start eating bran cereal, or eat more salad with lunch and dinner daily. I also tell them to keep some over-the-counter fiber constipation remedies around made with psyllium or methylcellulose, which can be taken regularly and are safe. Also, Metamucil has come out with capsules that include calcium in them. Having extra calcium is useful in pregnancy, and if you don't already own other calcium supplements, this is a good way to have fiber without having to drink a large glass of a mixture.

Apple pectin is helpful in pregnancy for constipation, so eating an apple a day is certainly a good idea. Prune juice and prunes are excellent for constipation. Over-the-counter products such as docusate sodium have not been found to be harmful in pregnancy, but people do become dependent on over-the-counter constipation remedies, so I definitely recommend trying natural remedies first.

Vitamin C and magnesium are also supplements that, when taken in high amounts, cause loose stools. So I definitely recommend taking the upper limits recommended for pregnant woman if she has a problem with chronic constipation: vitamin C, up to 2000 mg per day, and magnesium, up to 350 mg per day. If higher dosages are warranted, please consult with your physician.

Make sure that you are on an essential fatty acid supplement. Make sure that you are taking your prenatal vitamins regularly, because constipation can block the proper absorption of nutrients, resulting in vitamin and mineral deficiencies. If you have definitely isolated iron as the cause of your constipation, be aware that almost all prescription prenatal vitamins and most over-the-counter prenatal vitamins do contain iron; you might be able to find a prenatal vitamin without iron in a health food store. GNC does have a prenatal vitamin formula without iron. Ginger (which you may have from a previous recommendation or another recommendation somewhere in this book), stimulates the digestive system and eases passage of food through the intestine. You can eat raw ginger. Ginger comes in teas and capsules, also. In case you do not prefer prunes, figs are also an excellent natural laxative. One can also go the health food store and get some barley juice or wheat grass in order to increase one's consumption of chlorophyll, which eliminates toxins and bad breath.

If you need to use an enema, I recommend a soap-suds enema or a plain-water enema using purified water. The over-the-counter salt-containing enemas are not what I prefer for pregnant women to use; they can cause fluid shifts in the body and can also cause hypernatremia, which is not a good result even if you are not a pregnant woman but certainly in pregnancy it should not be used without a doctor's supervision. If constipation is a chronic problem, make sure you consult with your physician to rule out the possibility of an obstructive lesion, and certainly present immediately to your doctor if you note blood in your feces. Another note about constipation: Many people are on iron and calcium, both of which can be associated with constipation; however, to remedy constipation, the first thing that some people might do is eliminate these two things. This is not the first thing I would suggest. I would first try to increase both fluid and fiber intake, and regularly take products with psyllium or eat high-fiber cereal. If you remain on your supplements and increase your water and fiber and your constipation is relieved, this is a good plan.

Depression

If you have already been diagnosed with depression and are on an antidepressant, I do not recommend discontinuing that antidepressant without first consulting with your physician. Many of the vitamins that I recommend can be taken in conjunction with the medicine you are already on. If you feel that you need to harm yourself or someone else, please seek professional help immediately and do not simply rely on the vitamins. For those of you who have not been diagnosed with depression but are feeling sad or melancholy or have had a very sad event happen, it would be reasonable to start taking supplements after you speak to your medical doctor if the two of you decide that medications are not appropriate or essential at this time. Symptoms of depression include chronic fatigue, sleep disturbances, changes in appetite, headaches, backaches, digestive disorders, restlessness, irritability, quickness to anger, loss of interest or pleasure and hobbies, and feelings of worthlessness and inadequacy.

Foods greatly influence the brain's behavior. A poor diet, especially one with a lot of junk food, is a common cause of depression.

The levels of brain chemicals called neurotransmitters, which regulate our behavior, are controlled by what we eat, and neurotransmitters are closely linked to mood. The neurotransmitters most commonly associated with mood are dopamine, serotonin, and norepinephrine.

For depression, I recommend the following:

- B-complex. Signs of low B vitamin tissue levels are mood changes and fatigue.
- Magnesium supplementation, up to 350 milligrams per day.
- Inositol, 1 gram, twice per day
- SAMe as directed on the bottle
- Fish Oil as directed on the bottle
- Pantothenic Acid, 100–500 milligrams per day

Do not take the SAMe if you have been diagnosed with manic depressive disorder or take prescription antidepressants.

Diabetes

Diabetes is a result of problems with the pancreatic hormone insulin. Insulin controls the amount of glucose, or "sugar in the blood," and the rate at which is absorbed into the cells. The cells need glucose to produce energy. In people with diabetes, glucose builds up in the bloodstream instead of being taken into and used by cells; this leads to hyperglycemia, which is abnormally high levels of glucose in the blood. Eventually, hyperglycemia leads to damaged blood vessels, which in turn may cause eye disease, heart disease, and kidney disease.

Gestational diabetes is a form of the condition that develops during pregnancy and affects about 4% of pregnant women. Hormonal changes during pregnancy can affect the body's resistance to insulin. There are factors secreted by the placenta that can cause this. Most often this condition disappears after delivery, but it seems to be a sign that the woman is more likely to develop type 2 diabetes in later life. If you are on insulin or some other prescription remedy for your diabetes, please do not discontinue this medication in order to try nutritional supplementation, and do let your doctor know if you are taking nutritional supplements to lower your blood glucose. Your insulin or other medications may need to be adjusted but in general they are safe to take together; however, more intense monitoring should be done.

Brewer's yeast with added chromium can help lower blood sugar levels.

Biotin and inositol improve the metabolism of glucose. A B-complex vitamin could help you supply this biotin, because B-vitamins work best when taken together.

Zinc should be taken at 40 mg, which is the maximum in pregnancy. Deficiency of zinc has been associated with diabetes.

Low readings of magnesium are often found in people with diabetes, and magnesium supplementation could be beneficial. A dosage of 350 mg in pregnancy is the maximum.

Vitamin A is an important antioxidant needed to maintain the health of the eyes, because vision can deteriorate in diabetes.

Quercetin also helps protect the membranes of the lens of the eye that can occur as a result of high glucose levels.

Bilberry is an herb that may be beneficial for diabetes.

Ginsing tea is believed to lower the blood sugar level.

Fiber is recommended in diabetics to help the elimination process.

In women who are not pregnant, losing excess weight improves blood sugar levels. Weight loss is not recommended in pregnancy, but it is important to follow your diabetic diet and use alternatives to sugar to sweeten things, or learn to enjoy things unsweetened. High fiber lowers insulin levels and protects against obesity and heart disease, which is common in diabetics.

Eczema

Eczema is an inflammatory condition of the skin that can produce scaling, flaking, thickening, weeping, crusting, color changes, and, often, itching. Several conditions can exacerbate eczema. Candidiasis and food allergies are commonly experienced by pregnant woman and might cause an exacerbation of eczema. Pregnancy does not necessarily make eczema worse or better. Some of the prescription medications used to treat eczema have not been around very long and haven't been taken by many pregnant women for very long amounts, so their effects are unknown. Therefore, vitamin remedies certainly are worth trying, as follows:

- Vitamin A: Needed for smooth skin and aids in preventing dryness. Usually the amount in your prenatal vitamin is helpful. This is usually as beta carotene; one could take extra vitamin A, especially if it is combined with a vitamin C&E formula.
- Vitamin C: Useful because it inhibits inflammation and stabilizes cell membranes.
- Vitamin E: Relieves itching and dryness. If your prenatal vitamin contains beta carotene and you find an AC&E formula over-the-counter in which the A is less than 5000 international units daily and the vitamin E is 400 international units daily, this should be helpful.
- Essential fatty acids: Useful in pregnancy anyway. Make sure that you are on the supplement or prenatal vitamin that adds this supplement to the packaging, because it promotes lubrication of the skin.
- Zinc: Also useful. The maximum safe level in pregnancy is 40 milligrams. It aids healing and enhances immune function.
- Vitamin B-complex: Needed for healthy skin and proper circulation. It aids in the reproduction of all cells to help you make healthy new cells. Use a high-stress, yeast-free formula. If you do have a yeast infection, get this under control and try to control all other infections in the body, because once your immune system is busy attending to other things, your eczema can sometimes worsen at this time.

It is also good to avoid foods that sometimes people are allergic to and see whether certain foods are exacerbating your eczema. It is a good idea to avoid eggs, peanuts, soy foods, and wheat and dairy products. Remove these items one at a time from your diet and see whether you note any improvement. Also, sugar, strawberries, chocolate, white flour, fats, fried foods, and processed foods contain many things that increase inflammation. You can also try a gluten-free diet for six weeks and then add gluten-containing foods back into the diet one at a time and see whether the condition changes. A gluten-free diet is often of therapeutic benefit in controlling dermatitis.

Chamomile can be taken internally or used externally to soothe the skin. It may reduce inflammation.

<u>Fatigue</u>

A common complaint, especially in early pregnancy, is fatigue. There are many causes of persistent fatigue, which is different from being simply tired from exercising or a heavy workload. Fatigue may indicate a serious medical disorder such as anemia, diabetes, heart disease, cancer, chronic fatigue, or some dysfunction, hypothyroidism, or an infection. If you are extremely fatigued, please consult your physician. If nothing serious is found, supplementation may be in order. Some chronic, everyday problems may also cause significant ongoing fatigue such as stress, dietary imbalance, food allergy, nutritional deficiency, environmental toxicity, low blood sugar, and low-grade depression. Sometimes the problem is as simple as a lack of adequate exercise, or boredom. General things that can reduce fatigue include eating properly, exercising, and reducing emotional stressors. In addition to your prenatal vitamin, I recommend chromium, 200 micrograms, and magnesium (a maximum of 350 mg in pregnancy). Some studies utilizing oral magnesium and potassium aspartate found that between 75 and 91% of the nearly 3,000 patients studied experienced a decrease in fatigue during treatment; in contrast, the number of patients responding to placebo was between 9 and 26%. The beneficial effect was usually noted after only four or five days, but sometimes 10 days were required. Vitamin C up to 2000 mg is safe in pregnancy. Vitamins A and E are also antioxidants and powerful free-radical scavengers that protect the cells and enhance immune function and can help fatigue that is secondary to environmental causes. Vitamin B-complex contains the B vitamins that are essential for an increase in energy level and maintenance of normal brain function. If you have fatigue in addition to anemia taking an iron supplement and reading the anemia section is also helpful in conjunction with is already been noted. Chocolate, soft drinks, caffeine and highly processed food sugar highs can also create a low, what goes up must come down also these food deplete the body of magnesium which leads to fatigue. Do not smoke and avoid second hand smoke as this can make symptoms worse. Essential fatty acids are also good supplements, zinc up to 40 mg in pregnancy can be used.

Gallstones

Abnormal concentration of bile acids, cholesterol, and phospholipids in the bile can cause formation of gallstones. It is estimated that 20 million Americans have gallstones. In fact, one in 10 people have gallstones without even knowing it. If a stone is pushed out of the gallbladder and lodges in the bile duct, this can cause nausea, vomiting, and pain in the upper-right abdominal region. These symptoms often arise after the individual has eaten fried or fatty foods. If the gallbladder becomes inflamed, this condition requires immediate treatment. If left untreated, it can be life threatening. If you experience pain in your upper abdomen that lasts for more than an hour, you need to notify your doctor for directions on how to proceed. If you have known stable gallbladder disease, there are some additional supplements that may be of help to you:

- Essential fatty acids: Needed for repair and prevention of gallstones.
- Vitamin B-complex: Recommended because all B vitamins are necessary for proper digestion.
- Inositol: Should be used because it is important in cholesterol metabolism and liver and gallbladder function.
- Vitamin C: Maximum dose is 2000 milligrams in pregnancy; vitamin C deficiency can lead to gallstones.
- Vitamin D-3: 400 international units daily. This is normally already provided in your prenatal vitamin. Additional supplementation should not be necessary if you are able to take your prenatal vitamin daily. This supplement is important because gallbladder malfunction interferes with vitamin D absorption.

If you have an attack or accidentally eat something fatty and start to feel discomfort, drink one tablespoon of apple cider in a glass of apple juice. This should relieve the pain quickly. If the pain does not subside, call your physician for directions on how to proceed.

Pregnancy is not the optimal time for gallstone and gallbladder interventional treatment, such as surgery and lithotripsy. Following a diet consisting of 75% rough foods including applesauce, eggs, yogurt, cottage cheese, and beets and consuming as much apple, pear, and beet juice as possible will help to minimize the discomfort and complications of gallbladder disease.

Gastroenteritis

Gastroenteritis can be caused by a virus and passed from person to person in a household or can be caused by food contaminants. If the symptoms persist for more than 48 hours, please see your physician to make sure that it is not hepatitis or a symptom of some other more serious disease, but if everyone in your household is sick and it lasts for less than 24 hours, remedies can be tried at home after consultation with your physician. Symptoms include nausea, vomiting, abdominal cramps, diarrhea, and, occasionally, chills and low-grade fever. If you are unable to keep food or the supplements I recommend down, or you see blood in your diarrhea when you're vomiting, or you become dehydrated, please contact your physician for further instructions.

- Vitamin C, up to the maximum of 2000 mg in pregnancy, detoxifies the body and aids in removing bacteria and toxins.
- Acidophilus, taken as directed on the label, replaces essential intestinal bacteria.
- Fiber removes bacteria that have attached themselves to the colon walls and prevents the bacteria from entering the bloodstream. This action reduces symptoms and speeds recovery. One can buy over-the-counter fiber, such as any product containing psyllium. If you suspect food poisoning, call your regional poison control center immediately. Poison control centers can be reached 24 hours per day and can provide you with up-to-date information regarding treatment.

Headache

Virtually everyone gets a headache at one time or another. In the first trimester of pregnancy, headache is extremely common. Sometimes it's due to hormonal changes, sometimes to the fact that people have nausea and morning sickness and are not eating as much as usual, which causes a headache. Other common causes of headaches include: stress, tension, anxiety, allergy, constipation, coffee consumption, dehydration, eyestrain, hunger, sinus pressure, and muscle tension. Migraines result from a disturbance in the blood circulation in the head. Headache experts estimated that 90% of all headaches are tension headaches and 6% are migraines. Headaches can also be a sign of an underlying health problem. People who suffer from frequent headaches may be reacting to certain foods and food allergies such as wheat, chocolates, monosodium glutamate, sufites (which are used in restaurants on salad bars), sugar, hotdogs, lunch meats, dairy products, nuts, citric acids, fermented foods, cheeses, sour cream, yogurt, vinegar, or marinated foods. Other possibilities to consider are anemia, bowel problems, brain disorders such as tumors, hypoglycemia, sinus disorders, toxic overdose of vitamin A, vitamin D deficiency, and diseases of the eye, nose and throat. Dehydration can also cause headaches. If you are suffering from new onset headaches, don't assume that it is just the normal part of pregnancy; make sure to speak to your physician and are evaluated to rule out an associated disorder. Also discuss with your physician your plans for supplementation. The recommended supplements are as follows:

- Bromelain
- Calcium and magnesium: Magnesium can be used up to 350 mg a day and can be taken in divided doses; calcium can be taken in divided doses between 1200 and 1500 mg per day. There is considerable evidence that low magnesium levels trigger both migraine and tension headache. In individuals with low magnesium levels, magnesium supplementation has been shown to produce excellent results in double-blind studies.
- Glucosamine sulfate: This is a natural alternative to aspirin and other nonsteriodal B-complex vitamin, use the yeast free formula.
- Vitamin C: This vitamin helps the detrimental effects of pollution and age. (use a buffered form).
- Vitamin E: Improves circulation. Start with 400 international units daily.

- Chamomile: Relaxes muscles and soothes tension; use a hot towel to relax your neck and shoulder muscles.

If you feel that your headache may be due to allergies or sinuses, please refer to both of those sections in this book after proper diagnosis by your doctor. Headaches or migraines follow the same supplementation regimen.

- Essential fatty acids are among the list of things that can be taken to help a headache.

There have a been a few case reports of Ginger being helpful in migraine headaches, but this application has not been supported by a formal clinical trial. However, during pregnancy, if your headaches are related to your morning sickness, or if you are having nausea, vomiting, or loss of appetite that are common in early pregnancy, ginger is something that you can try to relieve your headache. It is available as fresh ginger, in capsules, and as tea, and in ginger ale.

SamE has been shown to be a benefit and treatment of migraine headaches. The benefit arises gradually, and long-term treatment is required for therapeutic effectiveness.

One hypothesis on why migraines headaches develop asserts that it is caused by a reduction of energy production within the cell of blood vessels. Because riboflavin has the potential to increase production, it was thought that it might have preventive effects against migraines. A few preliminary studies have shown excellent results. In one double-blind study, riboflavin or a placebo was given for three months to 55 patients with a history of migraine headaches. Riboflavin was shown to be superior to placebo in reducing attack frequency and duration. The proportion of patients who improve to at least 50% was 59% for the Riboflavin group and only 15% for the placebo group. I recommend a B-complex that includes riboflavin.

Hemorrhoids

Hemorrhoids, otherwise known as piles, are varicose veins in the lining of the anus either near the beginning of the anal canal; internal hemorrhoids are located at the anal opening, but external hemorrhoids are the ones that are most uncomfortable. Sometimes the internal hemorrhoids protrude outside the anus; these are called prolapsing hemorrhoids. The symptoms are as follows: a swelling or soft lump at the anus, sometimes accompanied by pain and itching; passing mucus after a bowel movement; streaks of bright-red blood on the toilet paper or in the stool. The water in toilet may also be reddish from blood. Some of the causes are constipation, excessive straining during bowel movements, sitting too long on hard surfaces, a sedentary lifestyle, eating too many sweets and not enough fiber, and the weight changes associated with pregnancy, which can cause pressure that exacerbates hemorrhoids. Much of the advice in this hemorrhoids section is similar to the advice in the constipation section with a couple of additions but s I noted previously, magnesium and vitamin C, both of which if taken in high enough doses can cause loose stools, should be taken at the upper limits recommended in pregnancy, which is 350 mg for magnesium and 2000 mg for vitamin C. Vitamin B-complex is recommended because all B vitamins are vital for digestion. Improved digestion results in reduced stress on the rectum.

Fresh aloe vera gel applied directly to the anus has properties similar to aspirin. It can relieve pain and soothe the burning sensation.

Witch hazel is helpful because of its astringent properties. Witch hazel pads can be found at a pharmacy and witch hazel also comes in a bottle. If purchased in this form, it can be applied to a cotton ball and placed externally.

If your hemorrhoids are accompanied by constipation, please see the constipation section and follow these remedies. Also, warm sitz baths are soothing and beneficial. If your hemorrhoids are accompanied by bleeding, sometimes you should evaluate the toilet paper you are using. Try to avoid using rough toiler paper. Use moistened toilet paper or baby wipes instead.

For oral supplements, oxerutin, which is a bioflavonoid, 1000 mg daily, is reportedly helpful for hemorrhoids. Avoid excess caffeine because it can cause excess water loss, which is not advantageous.

Herpes Type 1 and Type 2

Herpes Type 1 causes cold sores and Type 2 causes genital herpes. Genital herpes is very common. One in every five persons over the age of 12 have it, although more than half never develop serious symptoms. More than 45 million Americans in total have it. A mild tingling and burning in the vaginal area may be the first sign of genital herpes in women. Within a matter of a few hours, blisters develop around the rectum, clitoris, cervix, and in the vagina. Painful urination could be a symptom during this episode. Herpes during pregnancy, if the outbreak happens around the time of delivery, is a virus that can cause infection in the baby, which can be very serious. Most doctors would recommend a cesarean section if the outbreak were to occur at this time. There are prescription medications available to decrease the frequency and severity of outbreaks. If you are on these medications, please do not discontinue them without discussing it with your physician. However, as far as vitamin and supplement support is concerned, if you have a partner with herpes and you have yet to experience the symptoms, it is a good idea to take supplements to improve your resistance. In early pregnancy, if you are not already on the prescription medications that are used to decrease the frequency and severity of outbreaks, you could try the vitamin supplements to see whether doing so results in any improvement.

The first important supplement is beta 1,3-d-glucan, which is useful for treating any bacterial, viral, or fungal disease. It stimulates the activity of macrophages, which are immune cells that surround and remove invading microorganisms and cellular debris. Use as directed on the label.

Regularly take your multivitamin as it has vitamin A or beta-carotene which are important for healing. Other recommended supplements are the following:

- Vitamin B-complex: Combats the virus and helps to keep it from spreading.
- Vitamin C: Up to 2000 mg daily is needed to prevent sores and inhibit the growth of the virus.
- Zinc, up to the maximum of 40 mg per day in pregnancy, boosts immune function. For herpes around your mouth, use the zinc lozenges
- Essential fatty acids: Useful for cell protection.

- Vitamin E: The use of 200–800 international units per day is important in healing and prevents the spread of the infection.

Enhancement of the immune status is a key to prevention and control of herpes; many people note that stress exacerbates their outbreaks. Some women get it monthly during their menstrual cycle. Sometimes people will get it more frequently in pregnancy because this is a stressful time. Taking vitamins can help support the immune system and decrease the outbreaks. The fewer outbreaks you have, the less of the chance you have of spreading it to your partner. Something than can be used topically to soothe the lesions of cold sores and genital herpes is lemon balm. It contains components that exert activity against the herpes simplex virus. In Germany, some clinical studies have shown positive effects. It promotes healing of the herpes blisters much more quickly than normal. The control group receiving other topical creams had a healing period of ten days while the group receiving the lemon balm cream was completely healed within five days. The lemon balm cream should be applied 2–4 times a day during an active recurrence. Detailed toxicology studies have demonstrated that lemon balm is extremely safe and suitable for long-term use. However, do not take this balm internally during pregnancy.

Homocysteine, Elevated Levels

Homocysteine is an amino acid that is produced in the body in the course of methionine metabolism. Under normal circumstances, we convert homocysteine into other harmless amino acids with the help of three B vitamins: folate, B6, and B12. When this conversion doesn't occur rapidly enough, due to a deficiency of B vitamins or a genetic defect, homocysteine can accumulate in the blood. High levels of homocysteine can damage the blood vessel walls and promote the buildup of cholesterol deposits. Getting the right amounts of the B vitamins is an important way to keep your blood homocysteine at a healthy level. This amino acid has been the focus of increasing attention in recent years because high levels of homocysteine in the blood are associated with an increased risk of cardiovascular disease. Further, it is known that homocysteine has a toxic affect on cells lining the arteries, makes the blood more prone to clotting, and promotes the oxidation of low-density liproproteins, which is LDL, the bad cholesterol, which makes it more likely that cholesterol will be deposited as plaque in the blood vessels. Some people do have a genetic defect known as a deficiency in the methyltetrahydrofolate reductase gene, which decreases their ability to use folic acid. A person could also have a deficiency of vitamin B-6, B-12 or folate, which can prevent homocysteine from converting rapidly enough. As a result, high levels of the amino acid accumulate in the body, damaging cell membranes and blood vessels and increasing the risk of cardiovascular disease, particularly atherosclerosis. In my patients with a deficiency of the methyltetrahydrofolate reductase gene, MHTFR, I add Folgard, which contains folic acid and B-12, to their regimen. It is possible to obtain this product over the counter. Folic acid comes in 800 micrograms over the counter and vitamins B-6 and B-12 also come individually over-the-counter; they can also be purchased as a complex. If you do have the deficiency of this gene, your doctor can usually prescribe a regimen to maximize these vitamins. Make sure that you continue this regimen, because MHTFR deficiency is a genetic defect and does not go away.

Inflammatory Bowel Disease

Chronic Inflammatory Bowel Disease includes Crohn's Disease and ulcerative colitis. Ulcerative colitis is a chronic disorder in which the mucous membranes lining the colon become inflamed and develop ulcers causing bloody diarrhea, pain, gas, bloating and, at times, hard stools. The colon muscles then have to work harder to move these hardened stools through the colon. Crohn's Disease is an inflammatory bowel disorder of unknown origin. It usually affects the lowest portion of the small intestine but can occur in other parts of the digestive tract, from the mouth to the anus. Crohn's disease causes inflammation that extends deep into the lining of the intestinal wall, frequently causing cramping, abdominal wall, diarrhea, rectal bleeding, loss of appetite, and weight loss. It can become better or worse during pregnancy. Crohn's disease can be difficult to diagnose because its symptoms are very similar to those of other intestinal disorders, particularly ulcerative colitis. My advice to patients who have either of these diseases, which are very rare, is identical regarding supplementation that is considered safe during pregnancy. Iron is usually depleted in people with chronic inflammatory bowel disease. It is not necessary to take if anemia has not been diagnosed, but in both ulcerative colitis and Crohn's disease, anemia can be present. If this is documented, blackstrap molasses or carbonyl iron are the gentlest forms to take. Other helpful supplements are the following:

- B-Complex: Use a hypo-allergenic formula. B-complex is needed for the constant supply of new cells. Sometimes injections are warranted during an active flare-up.
- Acidophilus: Used to replenish gut flora.
- Bromelain: Used to breakdown protein and assist digestion. The acidophilus will replace the healthy bacteria needed for good colon function.
- Omega-3 fatty acids: Needed for repair of the digestive tract and reduces inflammatory processes. Studies have shown that essential fatty acids may reduce Crohn's symptoms and aid in maintaining remission.
- Calcium and magnesium supplementation: Important because malabsorption of these essential minerals is a problem in these conditions. Calcium is also needed for the prevention of cancer, which may occur due to constant irritation.
- Vitamin C: Up to 2000 mg for a pregnant woman is needed for immune function and the healing of mucous membranes. Use a buffered type.
- Zinc: Needed for immune system and for healing. Do not exceed 40 mg daily.
- Slippery elm: Particularly useful in patients diagnosed with Crohn's Disease.

Gastrointestinal disorders can impair selenium absorption; supplement with 60 micrograms in pregnancy.

Insomnia

Trouble sleeping, either falling asleep or staying asleep, is a common problem that affects everyone at some time in different points in a pregnancy. It can be especially bothersome right before the baby comes. There are different things one can try as a means to improve sleep habits. A relaxing 15-minute hot bath with two cups of Epson salt before bed can be useful. Avoid stimulants prior to going to bed—coffee, tea, or cola—for 2–3 hours. Avoid large meals before bed but do eat a light snack of something healthful if you are hungry, such as some nuts or some vegetable sticks. Consider a noise machine that plays nature sounds. Do not smoke before bed because nicotine is a stimulant. Get regular daily exercise but don't do it right before bed because doing so could keep you awake. In your general diet, try to avoid coffee, sugar, chocolate, and alcohol. Avoid taking too many of your regular supplements before bed, including vitamin C. The supplements that one should take before bed include:

- Calcium, which is absorbed very well at night even though one can take divided doses throughout the day. It is good to take before bedtime.
- Magnesium supplements are good to take at night also.

If you are on extra vitamin B or a B-complex, try to take that in the mornings so that it does not keep you awake at night. Also a cup of tea at bedtime, such as chamomile tea, could be useful. Foods high in tryptophan can be useful. If you need a snack before bed, bananas, dates, figs, milk, tuna, turkey, whole grain crackers, or yogurt are good. Eating a half of a grapefruit at bedtime also helps. Avoid foods that contain tyramine before bed; it increases the release of norepinephrine, which is a brain stimulant. Foods that contain tyramine are bacon, cheese, chocolate, eggplant, ham, potatoes, sauerkraut, sugar, sausage, spinach, tomatoes and wine (the last of which you should not be drinking during pregnancy anyway).

Irritable Bowel Syndrome

This is one of the most common digestive disorders seen by physicians. It is estimated that about one in five adult Americans have symptoms of irritable bowel syndrome, although fewer than half of them seek a physician's help for it. Twice as many women suffer from the condition as men. It is sometimes called intestinal neurosis, mucous colitis, and spastic colon. It usually affects people between the ages of 25–45. Many pregnant women, whether they know it or not, may be affected by this. In irritable bowel syndrome the normally rhythmic muscular contractions of the digestive tract become irregular and uncoordinated, which interferes with the normal movement of food and waste material and leads to the accumulation of mucous and toxins in the intestine. The accumulated material sets up a partial obstruction of the digestive tract, trapping gas and stools, which in turn causes bloating, distention, and constipation. Irritable bowel syndrome may affect the entire gastrointestinal tract, from the mouth through the colon. There are no physical signs of disease in bowel tissue with this disorder and its cause is unknown. Lifestyle factors such as stress and diet are sometimes reported to be the cause, as are food allergies. The symptoms of irritable bowel syndrome may include abdominal pain, loss of appetite, bloating, constipation, and/or diarrhea often alternating, flatulence, intolerance to certain foods, mucous in the stools, and nausea. Pain is often triggered by eating and may be relieved by a bowel movement. Because of the pain, diarrhea, nausea, and sometimes severe headaches and even vomiting. A person with irritable bowel syndrome may dread eating.

Whether or not an individual with irritable bowel syndrome eats normally, malnutrition may result because nutrients often are not absorbed properly. As a result, people with irritable bowel syndrome require as much as 30% more protein than normal, as well as an increased intake of minerals and trace elements, which can quickly be depleted by diarrhea. Many other diseases can be related to irritable bowel syndrome, including candidiasis, colon cancer, diabetes, gallbladder disease, malabsorption disorders, pancreatic insufficiency, ulcers, and parasitic infections. It is important to consult with your physician to rule out these other, more serious conditions before you start supplementing yourself for irritable bowel syndrome.

More than one hundred different disorders may be linked to the systemic effects of irritable bowel syndrome. One disorder that is linked in about 25% of adults with irritable bowel syndrome is arthritis. For irritable bowel syndrome, regular fiber is a good idea to keep your colon cleansed. Chamomile and ginger teas are good for irritable bowel syndrome. Avoid chamomile if you are allergic to ragweed. Slippery elm is another herb that is good to use in irritable bowel syndrome. Limit your consumption of gas-producing foods such as beans, broccoli, and cabbage if they cause any problems. You can use a vitamin B-complex. Make sure that it includes vitamin B-5, pantothenic acid. People with colon problems sometimes do not absorb B vitamins properly. Lactobacillus is good to replenish the friendly bacteria. Try to find a nondairy formula. Essential fatty acids are useful in protecting the intestinal lining. Zinc and Vitamin A are good supplements. Zinc can be used at up to 40 milligrams. If one already takes a prenatal vitamin that contains beta-carotene, that is sufficient. Peppermint tea is also soothing and useful in irritable bowel syndrome.

Kidney Stones

These are accumulations of mineral salts that can lodge anywhere along the course of the urinary tract and can be one of the most painful of all health ailments; in some people, they occasionally rival the pain of labor. Human urine is often saturated to the limit with uric acid, phosphates, and calcium oxalate. Normally, due to the secretion of various protective compounds and natural mechanisms that control pH of urine, these substances remain suspended in solution. However, if the protection compounds are overwhelmed or immunity becomes depressed, the substances may crystallize and the crystals may clump together, eventually forming stones large enough to restrict urinary flow. These stones can be jagged or smooth. Symptoms of kidney stones include: pain radiating from the upper back to the lower abdomen and groin, profuse sweating, frequent urination, pus and blood in the urine, odorous or cloudy urine, absence of urine formation, and sometimes chills and fever. An estimated 10% of Americans develop kidney stones at some point in their lives. There are more prevalent in the Southeastern United States than in other parts of the country. The reason for this is not known but it is theorized that the hot climate, which promotes dehydration, and/or regional dietary habits may be to blame. Kidney stones are ten times as common now as they were at the start of the twentieth century.

I will start with the simplest things before getting to what supplements to take. To maintain good kidney function, one should drink plenty of water, at least 64 ounces daily, which is eight,

8-ounce glasses of water. Pregnant women should improve upon this. If you live in a hot climate, you should be drinking even more. By far the single most important measure one can take to prevent kidney stones from forming is to increase water consumption. Water dilutes urine and helps prevent concentrations of the minerals and salts that can form stones. As a matter of fact, chronic dehydration is a major factor in kidney stone disease in 15–20% of people. Also drink unsweetened cranberry juice to help acidify the urine unless you are prone to the uric acid stones. If you do not like the taste of unsweetened cranberry juice, the pill form of cranberries can be taken. Drinking the juice of a fresh lemon in a glass of warm water the first thing each morning can help prevent stones from forming also. Use only distilled water for drinking and cooking. Avoid carbonated soft drinks.

The supplements that should be taken in kidney disease are as follows:

- Inositol: Has been proven in many studies to prevent and treat kidney stones.
- Magnesium: The maximum safe level in pregnancy is 350 milligrams. It reduces calcium absorption and can lower urinary oxalate, a mineral-salt common in kidney stones. Vitamin B-complex taken with magnesium reduces oxalate.
- Zinc: The maximum safe level in pregnancy is 40 milligrams. It is an important inhibitor of crystallization, which can lead to stone formation.
- Multivitamin complex: Your prenatal vitamin, hopefully.
- Extra Vitamin C: The maximum amount in pregnancy is 2000 milligrams. It acidifies urine, which is good because most stones will not form in acidic urine.
- Calcium: When you are taking your calcium supplement, take it only with food so that it will bind the oxalates in the food, making them unavailable for stone formation.
- Vitamin E supplement is also helpful.

Lupus or Positive Antinuclear Antibody Screen

Lupus is a chronic inflammatory disease that can affect many of the body's organs. It is an autoimmune disease, that is, it occurs when the immune mechanism forms antibodies that attack the body's own tissues. Many experts believe that it is due to an as-yet-unidentified virus. The disease was named lupus, which means wolf, because many people who got it developed a butterfly-shaped rash over the cheeks and nose that was considered to give them something of a wolf-like appearance. In fact, the rashes may appear elsewhere on the body such as chest, ears, hands, shoulders, and upper arms. Ninety percent of those who contract lupus are women. It usually develops between the ages of 15 and 35. I do not in my practice have a lot of pregnant women with lupus but I do have people who have different types of complaints that women with lupus have and also have a positive antinuclear antibody. My recommendation for people with lupus and people with the positive nuclear antibody and some of the features of lupus are the same. Also, the supplements in this section apply to people with the rheumatoid arthritis or test positive for rheumatoid arthritis factor. According to the American Rheumatism Association, four out of the following eight symptoms must occur, either at the same time or not, before a diagnosis can be made. However, even if I have a patient who does not meet the criteria of having four out of eight symptoms, but has enough vague symptoms that are similar to the complaints of people with lupus during pregnancy, I do recommend the same vitamin supplementation. The symptoms used in a diagnosis of lupus are as follows:

1. Abnormal cells in the urine
2. Arthritis
3. Butterfly rash on the cheeks
4. Low white blood cell count, low platelet count, or hemolytic anemia
5. Mouth sores
6. Seizures or psychosis
7. Sun sensitivity
8. The presence in the blood of a specific antibody that is found in 50% of people with lupus

Other symptoms that people with lupus can have include: abdominal and chest pains; blood in the urine; fatigue; hair loss; loss of appetite; low-grade fever; nausea; poor circulation in the fingers and toes; shortness of breath; vomiting; and weight loss. They can also have depression and headaches.

There is mounting evidence that fish oil supplementation may beneficially influence the course of treatment in patients with autoimmune diseases. The best studied of these is rheumatoid arthritis, for which double-blind studies have shown that fish oil supplementation is capable of producing significant clinical improvement in the amount of painful joints, inflammation, and pain. I would also recommend that people with positive antinuclear antibody or lupus take this supplement. Pregnant women, in general, even those who don't have any of these symptoms, should consider this supplement important.

Calcium and magnesium are also important supplements. In pregnancy, 1200 mg of calcium supplementation is standard, and for magnesium, the upper limit is 350 mg in pregnancy. These supplements are necessary for pH balance and for protection against bone loss due to arthritis. Other recommended supplments are as follows:

- Vitamin C, the maximum 2000 mg in pregnancy, aids in normalizing immune function.
- Zinc, the maximum 40 mg daily, aids in normalizing immune function, protects the skins and organs, and promotes healing.
- B-vitamin complex supplies commonly deficient nutrients. It can heal mouth sores, protect against anemia, and protect the skin tissues.
- Vitamin E is a powerful antioxidant that helps the body use oxygen more efficiently and promotes healing. An amount of 400–800 international units daily is good to take.
- Vitamin A is a potent antioxidant and free-radical scavenger needed for tissue healing. It is usually found in the prenatal vitamin. If not, beta-carotene, up to 10,000 international units a day, or vitamin A, 5000 international units a day, or a combination of the two, can be used.

Some lupus cases can be caused by medication. It is wise to review your list of medications with your physician. People with lupus can also have a false-positive blood test result for syphilis. I do recommend that people with the false-positive blood result for syphilis consider these vitamin supplements. Gluosamine sulfate is also a product that can be considered for someone with lupus, especially if the lupus has features of arthritis. It is also a good supplement to consider if your family has a strong history of arthritis, or if you have a positive antinuclear antibody or positive rheumatoid arthritis factor.

<u>Morning Sickness</u>

Morning sickness can occur in the morning, afternoon, or night. It may last all day. It is also referred to as nausea and vomiting of pregnancy, or, in severe cases, hyperemesis gravidarum. Good nutrition at least three months prior to pregnancy is the best way to minimize the occurrence of the symptoms, but you may want to consult your doctor for a prescription to alleviate severe cases. First try separating your solid and liquid food items. Sometimes people tolerate one or the other better, and if you eat and drink together, it all comes up. Drink something, wait an hour, and then try something such as dry cereal or toast. Peeled fruits are also good because the outside is the most likely to house agents that you may be sensitive to. Mild cases may respond to the following remedies:

- For morning sickness, ginger tea, fresh ginger or ginger capsules are useful.
- Peppermint tea can improve nausea.
- Vitamin B-6 supplementation is highly recommended. If you are able to take your prenatal vitamin, it already has between 10–40 milligrams of vitamin B-6, therefore an extra 25 milligrams two more times a day will keep you below the limit of 100 milligrams a day. Otherwise you can take between a total of 75–100 milligrams daily in divided doses.
- There's also a homeopathic remedy called Natrum Fos 6X, which is found to improve mild nausea and vomiting of pregnancy.

If you are able to tolerate no solids or liquids, please consult your physician. For people who have mild nausea and vomiting and are still able to tolerate most food and liquids, the preceding remedies may be appropriate after consultation with your physician.

Obesity

Obesity is defined as a state of being more than 20% above normal body weight or having a body fat percentage greater than 30% for women. A pregnant woman is not supposed to diet. We do not encourage weight loss in pregnant women at all; however, some women who have very bad eating habits before pregnancy do improve their eating habits and this can control their weight gain, which is good. Also, I encourage people to avoid as many empty calories as possible. People think that they are eating for two but if you think as you as number one and the baby as number two, baby should be about seven pounds, so that is really only one-tenth of you, or less. You should be eating for one and one-tenth, not two. By all means, eat more vegetables and eat some protein. If you are hungry you can generally follow the four-food group diet and eat a variety of foods, but when you get hungry do not increase your intake of cupcakes or ice cream or juices. I encourage people to increase their fluid intake—meaning water and milk—not fruit juices and soda. The actual normal amount of weight gain for an average-weight person is 25–35 pounds. For someone who is underweight, it is 40 pounds; for someone who is overweight, it is 15 pounds. For someone who gained much over 40 pounds in a previous pregnancy, I will have her keep a food diary and we evaluate what types of things can be replaced with more healthful foods.

The supplements I encourage in people who are concerned about their weight gain or who already are carrying extra weight are mainly to stabilize their blood sugar, because if you eat something very sweet, or drink some juice or eat a cupcake, you will be happy for a while but the sugar will be dissolved pretty quickly and your blood sugar can drop very quickly. This blood sugar drop often triggers another hunger signal, making people eat more. Depending on what's available, you might eat something else that's pretty quick and easy but not healthful, and these things frequently are high in calories. So if you are taking a supplement that stabilizes your blood sugar—chromium, for example—you might have time to react differently and get a healthier food item instead of feeling shaky and needing to eat something immediately that is close at hand. If your sugar is forced to drop gradually, you have a half-hour to an hour to actually plan something healthful and that might take longer to prepare, such as a salad, cut-up vegetables, or fruit; this approach is much better than grabbing pre-packaged candy and snacks. Decreasing the amount of juice that you drink and resisting the temptation of a cupcake, a doughnut or a bag of potato chips each day can add up to quite a few pounds at the end of the pregnancy that you didn't gain and that you don't have to lose later. The following items can help maintain healthful eating habits:

- Fiber: Keep psyllium husks around. Metamucil has a number of convenient packaging ideas. Benefiber is available in chewable tablets. Metamucil has calcium combined in its capsules. Psyllium capsules are good for higher low-blood sugar problems and gives a full feeling, cutting down hunger pains.
- Chromium: Using up to 200 mcg per day in pregnancy, chromium reduces sugar cravings by stabilizing the metabolism of simple carbohydrates.
- Essential fatty acids: If you are on a low-fat diet, it is good to provide yourself with additional essential fatty acids, which are needed by every cell in the body. They are also good for appetite control.
- Vitamin C: Using up to the 2000 mg maximum a day, vitamin C is necessary for normal glandular function. It also can speed up a slow metabolism, prompting it to burn more calories.
- Calcium: Calcium is involved in the activation of lipase, an enzyme that breaks down fats. Studies have also shown that people who have normal calcium levels lose weight faster than people who are not maximized on their calcium. This study was done on people who are exercising, and I do encourage all pregnant women to become active. Not marathon-runner active, but take 30-minute walks after dinner every day. If you are already active, check with your doctor to make sure that your activity is safe to continue. There are a number of pregnancy work-out videos on the

market; these are helpful if you prefer to exercise in your home and don't have time to go out or don't belong to a gym. If you have access to a pool, try walking through the water in the pool; this activity provides some extra resistance, and you are less likely to fall. Swimming, if you know how to swim, is safe in pregnancy. Exercise only if you do not have any other pregnancy-related problems, and please consult your physician before you begin any exercise program.
- Choline and inositol: Take as directed on the label; these help the body burn fat.
- A vitamin B-complex: Good for proper digestion.
Vitamin B-2, which is riboflavin, is required for efficiency in burning calories. Vitamin B-3 lessens sugar cravings. Vitamin B-6 boosts metabolism, so a B-complex vitamin is certainly an addition to the prenatal basic supplement that should be taken.
- Zinc: Up to 40 mg a day. Zinc enhances the effectiveness of insulin and boost immune function.

Preeclampsia

Preeclampsia is a disorder of pregnancy which includes features of hypertension, protein in the urine, and edema. For preeclampsia, several supplements have been studied, with mostly positive results. In addition to a prenatal vitamin, the following are recommended:

- Fish oil.
- B-complex tablet.
- Vitamin C: Upper limit of normal is 2000 milligrams.
- Vitamin E: Between 400–1000 international units.
- Calcium: 12–1500 milligrams.
- Magnesium: Upper limit is 350 milligrams.
- Zinc: Upper limit is 40 milligrams.

If you have a history of high blood pressure, have had preeclampsia in the past, or are very young or very old for a pregnant woman, whether a teenager or over the a[ge...] consider maximizing these supplements. Cal[cium...sup]plement because deficiency has been link[ed...] Essential fatty acids are important for ci[rculation and] blood pressure. Vitamin E improves he[art health and is a] blood-thinning agent. Vitamin C impro[ves...and] reduces blood-clotting tendencies. Magnesium deficiency has also been linked to high blood pressure. A selenium deficiency has been linked to heart disease, so supplementing with 200 micrograms daily can be beneficial. Vitamin B-complex is important for circulatory function and for lowering blood pressure. In pregnancy, do not take additional niacin except under the supervision of a physician. The upper limit of niacin in pregnancy is 35 milligrams. It is found in most prenatal vitamins. Inositol, 50 milligrams twice a day, has also been found to be of benefit.

Premature Labor

Premature labor occurs when a baby is born between the 20th and 37th week of gestation. A variety things can cause early delivery, including but not limited to: infections, uterine anomalies, and multiple gestations. These can be can be responsible for preterm rupture of membranes or preterm delivery. If one of these was the reason for your previous delivery, supplementation is still okay, but I would actually encourage it if you had an early delivery without a known reason. In addition to taking their prenatal vitamins, patients can ask their doctor about the following supplements:

- Vitamin C: For stabilization of the amniotic membrane, between 500 milligrams and 2000 milligrams per day.
- Calcium: 1200 milligrams is a good amount to be taken. There has not been conclusive evidence that calcium helps, but it has been studied. Also the reviews on magnesium are mixed but it is not harmful up to 350 milligrams per day along with your calcium.
- Zinc: Zinc has also been studied in small trials; take 15–40 mg per day.
- Omega-3 fatty acids: Low levels of dietary omega-3 fatty acid intake are thought to lead to increased prostaglandin

synthesis and preterm labor. In animal models, supplementation with omega-3 fatty acids offsets these effects.

Psoriasis

Psoriasis appears as patches of skin on the legs, knees, arms, elbows, scalp, ears, and back that are red or brown in color and covered with silvery-white scales. It often runs in families and the condition is linked to a rapid growth of cells in the skin's outer layer. These growths on the epidermis never mature. Whereas a normal skin cell matures and passes from the bottom level to the top in about 28 days, these abnormal cells form in about eight days, causing scaly patches. The condition is not contagious. The pattern is usually flare-ups and remission. Sometimes the condition improves in pregnancy and sometimes becomes worse in pregnancy, but the attacks can be triggered by stress, illness, injury and use of certain drugs.

In previous skin sections I have recommended vitamins A, C, and E, which are good for skin, of course. For your prenatal vitamin, your vitamin A should be in the form of beta-carotene, but there are over-the-counter antioxidant supplements that come in an A, C, and E formula. Take no more than 5000 international units of A or a formula containing no more than that and 400 international units of vitamin E.

Zinc, up to 40 milligrams per day, is good for immune system and skin healing. Of course, if your prenatal vitamin isn't one of those packaged already with an essential fatty acid supplement, make sure that you switch to one of those. It is also easy to obtain an essential fatty acid supplement from over-the-counter.

B vitamins are necessary for healthy cell growth, so a B-complex vitamin is also good. One tablespoon of lecithin twice a day is also recommended. Make sure that you are regularly taking your prenatal vitamin. Also, one can use emu oil, topically, for psoriasis. Chamomile tea is good to take internally and to place externally; aloe vera is also good to use externally. Vitamin E can be used topically.

Chamomile, aloe vera, and vitamin E can all be used to help soothe the itching so that one does not scratch and make it worse.

Fumaric Acid and citrus bioflavinoids are also useful in this condition. Omega 3 fatty acids should be used as directed; they contain ingredients that interfere with the production and storage of arachidonic acid.

Rash

Rash is a common complaint in pregnancy. We can come into contact with some sort of soap that irritates our skin or clothing that irritates our skin, but during pregnancy it definitely can be a sign of something more serious. If you do have a rash, please have your doctor examine it to make sure that it is not a symptom of an underlying disease or condition such as a liver disorder. However, if you discover this rash over the weekend before your doctor's office opens on Monday, you can try a couple of things that will not harm your evaluation. I encourage my patients to try the following:

- Essential fatty acid: If you are on a prenatal vitamin that does not contain this, you can get these supplements over-the-counter. Use them as directed on the bottle.
- Aloe vera: I usually advise my patients to use aloe vera topically. The plant is relatively easy to find and is relatively inexpensive. You can break a piece open and apply the liquid from the plant directly onto the rash. This frequently helps the rash resolve.
- Chamomile: If you have chamomile tea from one of my previous recommendations, you can use this tea to apply topically; it is very soothing to the skin.
- Vitamin E: If you have vitamin E capsules around, take the oil of a vitamin E capsule and rub it on your skin. Sometimes rashes are due to dryness, which makes you scratch and can lead to a rash. Sometimes vitamin E will add moisture back to your skin and stop the cycle of itching and scratching.

When you take your shower or bath, try to avoid using the same washcloth or sponge each time you shower, because bacteria and fungi can grow in these moist areas and could be the cause of your rash. You can even try to change your soap. I usually recommend oatmeal soap. Switching to other hypoallergenic skin care products can be helpful. There are some products in health food stores. If your rash is under your arms, deodorants made of crystals are available that do not cause irritation. Try to find things that are unscented.

Sciatica

Sciatica is an inflammation of the sciatic nerve that starts in the lower back and runs across the buttocks and into the leg, calf, and foot. Many pregnant women are plagued by this and it is frequently exacerbated by the position of the baby, which of course is difficult to change during the course of a pregnancy. The symptoms are any or all of the following: nagging, aching, tingling, and burning or numbness that can start or remain in the buttocks or travel the course of the sciatic nerve down the back of the thigh and the front of the foreleg. It is usually limited to one side. It may be sensitive to temperature changes and touch and may radiate down to the toes, causing a lump. Disc herniation is usually associated with lower-back pain and is often worse on bending backwards and better lying down. Some remedies for this are ice packs or wet heat. I recommend a high-fiber diet if you note that constipation is making your pain worse. Drink 6–8 glasses of bottled mineral water a day. Nutrients that should be taken are as follows:

- Calcium or magnesium: Natural muscle relaxants
- Thiamine
- B-complex 50
- Essential fatty acids: Good for the repair and flexibility of the muscles

Smoking Dependency

Every time a person smokes, he or she inhales more than 4,000 different chemicals, including nicotine. Nicotine, which is extremely addictive, increases the level of the pleasure-inducing brain chemicals, serotonin, dopamine, and norepinephrine. During pregnancy, the baby is inhaling these same toxic chemicals. Pregnancy is an excellent time to quit smoking. Smoking increases the risk of catching colds and lengthens the recovery time. Smokers tend to have more miscarriages, stillbirths, and premature deliveries. Their babies are often smaller and have more health problems than babies of nonsmokers. Infants whose mothers smoke both during pregnancy and after childbirth appear to be three times as likely to die of sudden infant death syndrome, or SIDS, as infants of nonsmokers.

Smoking has a detrimental effect on nutrition. Smokers break down vitamin C about twice as fast as nonsmokers. Other antioxidant vitamins are depleted as well. The nutrients and dietary suggestions that I make here are recommended to correct probable smoking-related deficiencies and damage while you work to kick the habit. Many over-the-counter products that contain nicotine are not recommended in pregnancy, but please work with your physician to see whether buproprion is an option if you need it. If you are smoking to relieve stress or because you're getting stressed-out, also consult the stress chapter in this book. If you are following the supplement recommendations, you will be taking quite a number of pills per day. My recommendation is that every time you would like to have a cigarette, find one of your pills and take it instead. This might delay your consumption of a cigarette for another hour or two and over the course of each day you will probably be smoking fewer cigarettes than you were before you were pregnant. As you get more accustomed to taking the vitamins and spacing them out by taking them at different times of the day, you will probably be exposing the baby to a lot less nicotine overall. So in addition to your prenatal vitamin, I recommend:

- Vitamin C, with bioflavinoids, up to 2000 mg per day is okay in pregnancy. Vitamin C is important to protect cells against cell damage, and cigarette smoking does cause a lot of cell damage; also, smoking drastically depletes the body of vitamin C.
- Vitamin E is another important antioxidant. It is also needed to protect the cells and organs from damage by the smoke. Use the d-alpha-tocopherol form. Start with a 200 international unit supplement. Up to 1000 international units is safe in pregnancy, but I recommend about 200–400 international units unless you are also using vitamin C for another condition.

- B-complex is necessary in cellular enzyme systems that are often damaged in smokers. It may also help you through stressful periods so that you will not feel the need to smoke as frequently.
- Vitamin A is very important. Most likely you are getting this from your prenatal vitamin, 5000 international units, but if you are using an ACE antioxidant preparation, it is okay to either have 5000 international units of vitamin A or an additional 5000 units of beta carotene.
- Zinc is important in immune function. Sometimes there is some zinc in your prenatal vitamin but it would be advisable to use a supplement to get you up to the 40 mg maximum.
- Make sure that you are taking selenium; 60 mcg is the maximum amount for pregnancy.

Smoking is also a factor in the development and progression of cervical dysplasia. Smoking may decrease folic acid levels, which increase homocysteine levels and thereby increases the risk of coronary heart disease, heart attacks, bone loss, and pregnancy problems. In addition to your prenatal vitamin or daily multivitamin, take folic acid, which should be in a vitamin B-complex.

Stress

The term *stress* refers to any reaction to a physical, mental, social, or emotional stimulus that requires a response or alteration to the way we perform, think, or feel. Almost everyone who has this book will be reading this section because whether we are under stress chronically or intermittently, most of us are under stress. Very few of us get to lie at home watching TV with servants fanning us all day long while we never have to move or think about anything. Many of us go to work or leave our houses or have children or spouses to attend to. There are bills to be paid, or things to study at school or to learn at work. Change is stressful, whether the change is good or bad. Worry produces stress. Indeed, stress is an unavoidable part of life.

Supplement number one is a B-complex vitamin. Others are as follows:

- Vitamin C supplement, 500 milligrams
- Zinc
- Fish oil
- Calcium and magnesium, which are usually lost during stress. A deficiency can result in anxiety, fear and hallucinations.
- Inositol
- SAMe
- Pantothenic Acid, 100–500 milligrams

A study from Germany showed that people who took 1000 milligrams of vitamin C per day dealt better with psychological stress than those who did not take the supplement. The upper limit of safety during pregnancy is 2000 milligrams. If one were to take this level of vitamin C and experience any side effects, most commonly diarrhea, one should keep decreasing the dose by 500 milligrams until a comfortable level is reached. Anywhere between 500–2000 milligrams of supplementation is acceptable.

For SAMe, do not take if you have manic depressive disorder or take prescription antidepressants.

The B vitamins are important in cases of stress. One can take B-complex 50 that is sold over-the-counter, or the supplements can be taken individually.

Calcium and magnesium are lost when stress is present. The limit of calcium that should be taken in pregnancy is 1200 mg. Make sure that you are getting this amount daily. It would also be good to get a supplement that contains calcium, magnesium, and zinc together because extra zinc is also good during times of stress. The upper limit of safety in pregnancy is 40 milligrams of zinc. Chamomile tea will help you sleep if the stress is causing insomnia. Stress often causes diarrhea and/or constipation, so an increased intake of fiber is warranted. The over-the-counter fiber products that contain psyllium or methylcellulose are safe for daily use.

Stretch Marks

Everyone dreads these, and once you have them, there currently is no technology to remove them. It is hoped that one day there will be. But for now, there are things you can do internally and externally to minimize their appearance. First, the recommended weight gain for pregnancy is 25–35 pounds for a person of normal weight, 15 pounds for someone who is overweight, and up to 40 pounds for someone is underweight. No matter what vitamins I give you or what skin cream you take, if you gain 100 pounds during your pregnancy, your skin will likely stretch, so controlling weight gain is very important. The type of supplements that one can take internally are as follows:

- Vitamin C: Helps with collagen.
- Essential fatty acids: Follow the instructions on your bottle.
- Zinc: Up to 40 milligrams are safe in pregnancy.

Externally, one could use a topical cream containing any of the following, alone but preferably in combination:

- Aloe vera
- Vitamin E
- Cocoa butter

Thyroid Disease

Hypothyroidism affects nearly 5% of the population, whereas hyperthyroidism affects 2%. The thyroid gland is the body's internal thermostat. If the gland secretes too much hormone, hyperthyroidism results, leading to symptoms such as the following: heart palpitations, nervousness, insomnia, hair and weight loss, protruding eyeballs, and hand tremors. If the gland secretes too little hormone, hypothyroidism results, leading to symptoms such as fatigue, constipation, inability to tolerate cold, fertility problems, dry skin, and weight gain. Your health provider can draw your blood to evaluate you for these conditions. Untreated hyperthyroidism or hypothyroidism can also cause pregnancy complications, so make sure that you do not discontinue these medications without consulting your doctor. I recommend that my patients take the following supplements in addition to their prescription medications:

- B-complex: Combats the elevated homocysteine levels often associated with hyperthyroidism.
- Antioxidants are beneficial, including:
  Beta Carotene
  Vitamin C—important in this stressful condition
  Vitamin E 400 IU
- Essential fatty acids: Use as directed.
- Selenium: This trace mineral is an important component of an enzyme that produces thyroid hormone T3. A pregnant woman needs 60 micrograms of selenium per day. Most American women eat between 113 and 220 micrograms of selenium per day. Therefore, most women get the selenium requirement from their diet. The exception to this is vegetarians, who do not consume meat and seafood, which are good sources of selenium.

Urinary Tract Infection

This section is applicable to people who have a history of bladder infections or kidney infections. If you think you have a bladder infection, please see your physician to treat it with antibiotics and then consult this book for nutritional support to prevent it from happening again. The infections are caused by bacteria that enter the urinary tract. Eighty-five percent of the time, the bacteria that is the culprit is called *Escherichia coli*, which is a bacteria that is normally found in the intestines. There are other causes that also cause burning upon urination, frequency of urination, or urgency, which is when you go to the bathroom because you feel as though you have to urinate but nothing comes out. These conditions occur more frequently in women than men because of the close proximity of the anus, vagina, and urethra in females and also because of the short length of the female urethra. This allows for relative easy transmission of bacteria from the anus to the vagina and urethra, and subsequently it ascends to the bladder. The first thing I recommend is that women wipe from front to back, not from the anus to the vagina, but from the opposite direction.

Sometimes in a urinary tract infection, the urine has a strong, unpleasant odor and may appear cloudy. A pregnant woman who has a bladder infection may complain of a lower abdominal pain and discomfort and think it's the baby but it might indeed be a bladder infection. The first thing I tell people with a history of urinary tract infections or kidney infections is to take cranberries. Cranberries contain several substances that are thought to be clinically effective in the treatment of urinary tract infections. These substances can be obtained by eating the actual fruit cranberry or in pills that are sold in your pharmacy in the vitamin section; also, you can find them in commercial cranberry juice. Unfortunately, most commercial cranberry juices contain a large amount of sugar, and you have to drink quite a bit of it for it to be effective. I instruct my patients to drink unsweetened cranberry juice if they can tolerate it, but a lot of them like cran-grape, cran-apple, and cran-peach, which are supplemented with sugar. Sugar promotes bacterial growth, so I actually prefer the pills. If you do have some unsweetened cranberry juice, you can dilute it with water to make it easier to drink. I also recommend extra vitamin C, which produces an antibacterial effect through the deacidification of urine (up to 2000 mg can be taken safely in pregnancy). If you are prescribed antibiotics for your urinary tract infection, it is a good idea to follow this treatment with a course of acidophilus to restore the healthy bacteria. Calcium and magnesium reduce bladder irritability, and of course you should be on your multivitamin and mineral complex or prenatal vitamin.

Yeast, recurrent

I have many patients who, even if prior to pregnancy they didn't have many problems with yeast, cannot seem to get rid of a yeast infection during their pregnancy. Chronic yeast can lead to fatigue, give symptoms of a food allergy or environmental sensitivity, and cause other miscellaneous complaints. Yeast, most commonly Candida, which is found in the vagina, feed on sugar. If the body's pH balance is upset for any reason, the friendly bacteria such as lactobacilli that normally metabolize sugars cannot thrive and do their job properly, and there is a risk of candida albicans flourishing in this sugar-rich environment. Some women find themselves with more yeast infections when they use oral contraceptives or during pregnancy. This is most likely due to the increase in the amount of sugar in the vagina induced by changing hormone levels. Sometimes the hormones of the placenta conflict with the insulin that you normally produce, which usually is adequate for you but now it takes you longer to process sugar and it stays in your blood stream longer, and you start excreting it through your skin, urine, and vagina. It can also be seen in your urine when a urinalysis is performed in the physician's office. For my patients who complain of chronic yeast , the first thing I do is not supplement them with vitamins but instead talk to them about their diet. I tell them to increase their vegetable and protein intake and decrease their carbohydrate intake. I encourage them to drink more water as opposed to fruit juices and really watch their carbohydrate intake. They'll go on a low-carbohydrate diet and eat the bare minimum of breads and pastas and definitely no muffins out of a package, or chocolate muffins and cupcakes and the like. These dietary changes have caused an improvement in many people. Additionally, however, I do recommend certain supplements, as follows:

- Acidophilus or lactobacillus: Take it as directed on the label. There are formulations that one can take by mouth and formulations that one can take by vagina.
- Essential fatty acids.
- Pantothenic acid: Up to 250 milligrams.
- Vitamin C: Builds up immunity and protects the body tissues from damage by the toxins released from the candida.
- Vitamin E .
- Selenium: 60 micrograms daily.
- Zinc: Can be supplemented up to 40 milligrams per day.

Another good thing to incorporate into your diet if you have chronic yeast is plain yogurt that contains live yogurt cultures. One can also apply natural, unprocessed, and unsweetened yogurt directly into the vagina. This can be soothing until other types of things work. Also, always consult with your physician, because sometimes burning and discharge that may have been present in a prior yeast infection now indicates something else, and other things should be ruled out and treated if present. Other things to avoid are yeast products and sugar, aged cheeses, alcohol, chocolate, fermented foods, and honey. Wear white cotton underwear because synthetic fibers lead to increased perspiration, which creates a hospitable environment for candida and traps bacteria.

Suggested Reading

The following texts and articles were also used as resources:

Anderson, R.A. et al. (1987) Effects of supplemental chromium on patients with symptoms of reactive hypoglycemia . *Metabolism, 36(4)*, 351–355.

Ashe, JR, Schofield FA, Gram MR.(1979) The retention of calcium, iron, phosphorus, and magnesium during pregnancy: the adequacy of prenatal diet with and without supplementation. *American Journal of clinical nutrition 32*,86–91.

Avron, J. et al. (1994) Reduction of bactericidal and pyuria after ingestion of cranberry juice. *JAMA 271*,751–754.

Balch, P. and Balch, J. (2000) *Prescription for Nutritional Healing.* New York: Avery.

Basu, J. et al. (1991) Plasma ascorbic acid and beta-carotene levels in women evaluated for HPV infection, smoking, and cervix dysphasia.*Cancer detection and prevention, 15*(3):165–170.

Beazley, D, Ahokas R, Livingston, J., Griggs, M., Sibai, BM., (2005) Vitamin

C and E supplementation in women at high risk for preeclampsia: a double-blind, placebo-controlled trial. *American Journal of obstetrics and gynecology Feb: 192* (2):520–1.

Beck, L. (2001) *The Ultimate Nutrition Guide for Women.*(1st ed.). New Jersey: John Wiley and Sons.

Butterworth, C. et al. (1982) Improvement in cervical dysphasia associated with folic acid therapy in users of oral contraceptives: *American Journal of clinical nutrition 35*:73–82.

Czeizel AE, Dudas, I. (1992) Prevention of the first occurrence of neural tube defects by preconception vitamin supplementation. *New England Journal of Medicine. 327*:1832–5.

Gorbach, S.L. (1990) Lactic Acid bacteria and human health. *Annals of medicine. 22* (1):37–41.

Hass, E. (1992) *Staying Healthy with Nutrition.* Berkeley, California: Celestial Arts.

Institute of Medicine. (1998) Food and Nutrition Board. Dietary Reference

Intakes. Washington, DC: National Academy Press.

Janson, M. (2000) *Dr. Janson's New Vitamin Revolution.* New York: Avery.

Lankford, T. (1994) *Foundations of Normal and Therapeutic Nutrition*, (2nd ed.). Albany, New York:Delmar Publishers Inc.

Leiberman, S. and Bruning, N. (2003) *The Real Vitamin and Mineral Book*, New York: Avery.

Mackerras, D. et al. (1999) Randomized double-blind trial of beta-carotene and vitamin C in women with minor cervical abnormalities. *British Journal of cancer 79*(9–10):1448–1453.

Mastroiacovo P, Mazzone T, Addis A, et al. (1999) High vitamin A intake in early pregnancy and major malformations: a multicenter prospective controlled study. *Teratology 59*:7–11.

McGregor JA, Allen KGD, Harris MA, et al. (2001) The omega-3 story: Nutritional prevention preterm birth and other adverse pregnancy outcomes. *Obstetric and gynecologic survey 56*(suppl): S1–S13.

Murray, M.(2002) *The Pill Book Guide to Natural Medicines.* New York: Bantam.

Olsen SF, Secher NJ, Tabor A, Weber T, Walker JJ, Gluud C.(2000) Randomized clinical trials of fish oil supplementation in high risk pregnancies. Fish oil Trials In Pregnancy (FOTIP) Team. *British Journal of obstetrics and gynecology 107*:382–395.

Pauling, L. (1976) *Vitamin C, the common cold, and the flu.* San Francisco: W.H. Freeman and Co.

Schoenen, J. et al. (1998) Effectiveness of high-dose riboflavin in migraine prophylaxis. A randomized controlled trial. *Neurology 50*(2):466–470.

Villar J, Repke JT. (1990) Calcium supplementation during pregnancy may reduce preterm delivery in high-risk populations. *American Journal of obstetrics and gynecology 163*: 1124–31.

Index

Allergies 34, 47, 48, 50, 57, 62, 63, 70
    food 48, 50, 57, 62, 70
    seasonal 47
aloe Vera 64, 80, 81, 86
antinuclear antibody 72 – 75
anemia 12, 14, 15, 17, 20, 25, 37, 46, 59, 62, 68, 73, 74
    iron deficiency 46
    pernicious 12
    sickle cell 14
anxiety 12, 38, 45, 48, 62, 85
arthritis 9, 13, 31 34, 38, 46, 70, 73- 75
    osteoarthritis 13
    rheumatoid arthritis 13
asthma 17-19, 34, 48
b complex 14, 45, 47, 48, 51, 56, 58-60, 62- 65, 68, 69, 71, 72, 78, 79, 80, 82, 84, 87
Beta-carotene 8, 15, 49, 52, 58, 71, 74, 80, 84, 87
bilberry 40, 57
bioflavonoids 83 will
Biotin 8, 9, 12, 57
brewer's yeast 13, 24, 57

Bromelain 9, 10, 47, 50, 62, 68
calcium 12, 19 – 24, 26 – 28, 33, 45, 51, 54, 55, 62, 68, 69, 71-72, 74, 77 – 79, 82, 85, 88, 92
    and magnesium 22, 45, 85
    and preeclampsia 21
    and weight control 77
    and vitamin D 22
    in prenatal vitamins 22
    overdose of 23
    sources of 92
Candida 37, 88, 89, 90
candidiasis 34, 57, 70
carpal tunnel 15, 49 – 50
celiac disease 20, 50 – 51
cervical dysplasia 11, 51, 52, 84
    and smoking 84
chamomile tea 45, 69, 80, 81, 85
    and sleep 85
choline 35, 44, 78, 95
chromium 23 – 25, of 57, 59, 76, 77, 93
    and diabetes 23
    sources of 24, 93

toxicity 25
common cold 17, 19, 32, 33, 41, 42, 43, 52
constipation 5, 7, 23, 26, 46, 53 – 55, 62 64, 70, 82, 86
Copper 9, 18, 25, 93
cranberry 40 – 41, 72, 88
depression 6, 10, 12, 15, 17, 23, 31, 34, 35, 36, 38, 55, 56, 74
   postpartum depression 38
   SAMe and, 38
diabetes 9, 13, 19, 23- 25, 27, 35, 36, 56
   gestational diabetes 56
E. coli 41
eczema 15, 31 32, 34, 57, 58
essential fatty acids 33 – 35, 48, 51, 58 – 60, 63, 68, 71, 77, 79, 82, 86, 87, 89, 92
   and Crohn's 68
fatigue 12, 27 – 28, 38, 45, 47, 55, 56, 59, 73, 86, 88
   chronic fatigue syndrome 27-28
   SAMe and, 38
fiber 19, 33, 51, 53 – 55, 57, 61, 70, 77, 82, 85, 90
   and constipation 55
   and diabetes 57
fish oil 34, 35, 45, 56, 74, 78, 85
Folic acid 5, 10, 11, 12, 19, 37, 38, 44, 46, 48, 51, 52, 67, 84, 93
   and cervical dysplasia 11
   and depression 11
   and homocysteine 84

   and neural tube defects 10
   and pernicious anemia 12
   preconception 10
gastroenteritis 61
ginger 42 – 43, 54, 63, 70, 75
   and irritable bowel 70
Gotu Kola 45
headache 6, 7, 12, 14, 23, 28, 38, 42, 45, 47, 52, 55, 61, 62, 63, 70, 74
   during pregnancy 61
   migraine headache 14, 38, 42, 62, 63
   tension headach e 28, 62
   types of 62
hemorrhoids 63 – 64
herpes 64 – 66
high blood pressure 14, 21, 27, 78, 79
   and essential fatty acids 79
   and preeclampsia 78
   and the selenium deficiency 79
homocysteine 10 – 11, 66, 67, 84, 87
hyperemesis gravidarum 75
hyperthyroidism 86
hypothyroidism 86

inositol 35 – 36, 45, 56, 57, 60, 72, 78, 79, 85
   and depression 36
   and diabetes 35, 36, 57
insomnia 27, 68, 85, 86
iodine 36

iron 5, 6, 9, 18, 19, 25, 26, 33, 37, 46, 47, 51, 53, 54, 55, 59, 68, 88, 90, 93
   absorption 26
   sources of 93
   vitamins without 54
irritable bowel syndrome 43, 53, 69, 70, 71
kidney infection 88
kidney stones 18, 20, 22, 28, 71, 72
lactate 36
lactobacillus acidophilus 37, 71, 89
liver extracts 37
lupus 34, 72 – 75
magnesium 9, 26 – 30, 45, 51, 54, 56, 57, 59, 62, 64, 68, 69, 72, 74, 78, 79, 82, 85, 88, 93
   and migraines 62
   deficiency of 27, 51
   sources of 93
morning sickness or 42, 50, 63, 75
Natrum Fos 6x 75
niacin 13, 79
niacinamide 13
obesity 57, 76
pantothenic acid 12, 13, 45, 56, 71, 85, 89, 113
peppermint tea 43 – 44, 71, 75
preeclampsia 18, 21, 28, 32, 78
   antioxidants and 18
   previous pregnancy and 21
preterm labor 80
psoriasis 31 – 32, 34, 80
psychosis 73

rash 47, 73, 81, 82
   and chamomile tea 81
   and vitamin E. 81
   butterfly rash 73
riboflavin 13, 14, 63, 78, 94, 108, 114
SAMe 38, 39, 45, 56, 63, 73, 81, 82, 85, 92
sciatica 82
seizures 73
selenium 30 – 31, 47, 49, 68, 79, 84, 87, 89, 95
   sources of 95
smoking 48, 52, 53, 82, 83, 84
   and cervical dysplasia 84
stress 4,6, 12, 27, 46, 48, 50, 58, 59, 62, 64, 66, 70, 80, 83, 84, 85
stretch marks 85
thiamine 82, 94
thyroid 8, 22, 26, 36, 49, 53, 59, 86
   hormone 26
urinary tract infection 40 – 41, 87, 88
vitamin A 8, 15 – 16, 20, 26, 46, 49, 54, 57, 58, 60, 65, 71, 74, 80, 84, 94
   sources of 94
vitamin B6 44
vitamin C 6, 8, 17 – 19, 26, 31, 45 – 48, 51 – 54, 57 – 62, 64, 65, 68, 72, 74, 77 – 79, 83, 85-89, 92, 95
   and adrenal function 79
   and collagen 86
   sources of 95

vitamin D 19 – 20, 22, 60, 62, 95
    sources of 95
vitamin E 20, 30, 31, 46, 51-52, 58, 62, 66, 72, 74, 78-81, 83, 86, 87, 89, 91
    and dryness 58
    and itching 58
    function 20
    topically 81
yeast 27, 51, 58, 62, 88, 89
    and oral contraceptives 88
    chronic 89
zinc 8, 25, 26, 31, 32, 33, 46, 47, 52, 57-59, 65, 68, 71, 72, 74, 78-80, 84, 85, 86, 89, 95
    and diabetes 57
    and immunity 84
    and iron deficiency 46
    sources of 95
zinc lozenges 32, 65